P9-CLR-908

ANXIETY
RELIEF

FOR

TEENS

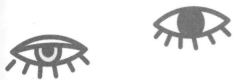

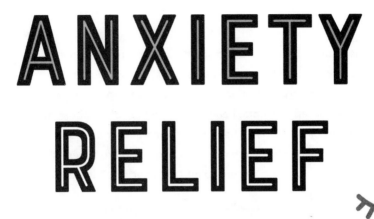

ANXIETY RELIEF FOR TEENS

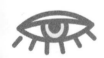

Essential CBT Skills and Mindfulness Practices to Overcome Anxiety and Stress

REGINE GALANTI, PhD

ZEITGEIST • NEW YORK

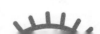

This book is designed to provide helpful information on the subjects discussed. It is not meant to be used for, nor should it take the place of, diagnosing or treating any medical conditions. Please consult a physician or mental health professional before adopting any exercises or guidelines. The publisher and author are not responsible for any specific health needs that may require supervision or consultation with a licensed and qualified healthcare provider.

Copyright © 2020 by Penguin Random House LLC

All rights reserved.

Published in the United States by Zeitgeist, an imprint of Zeitgeist™, a division of Penguin Random House LLC, New York.
penguinrandomhouse.com

Zeitgeist™ is a trademark of Penguin Random House LLC

ISBN: 9780593196649
Ebook ISBN: 9780593196700

Cover art © Faya Francevna/Shutterstock.com
Book design by Aimee Fleck
Interior art:
© Faya Francevna/Shutterstock.com
© Foxys Graphic/Shutterstock.com
© Pikovit/Shutterstock.com
Author photo © Leslie Renee Photography

Printed in the United States of America
5 7 9 10 8 6

First Edition

CONTENTS

INTRODUCTION 1

CHAPTER 1:
YOU CAN RETRAIN YOUR BRAIN 5

CHAPTER 2:
THE MIND-BODY CONNECTION 31

CHAPTER 3:
MANAGING DIFFICULT EMOTIONS 66

CHAPTER 4:
CHANGING YOUR THOUGHTS 89

CHAPTER 5:
CHALLENGING YOUR BEHAVIORS 115

CONCLUSION 166

APPENDIX 168

RESOURCES 171

REFERENCES 173

EXERCISE/SKILL INDEX 175

INDEX 176

ACKNOWLEDGMENTS 185

ABOUT THE AUTHOR 186

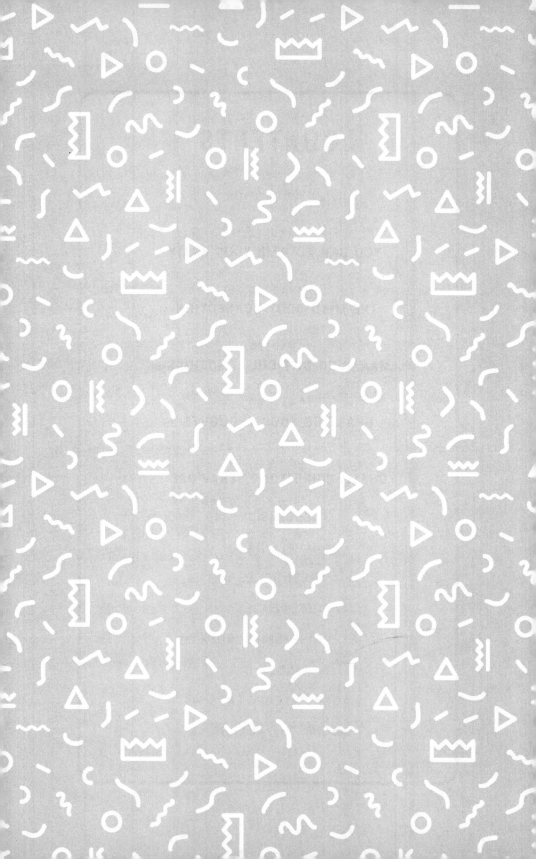

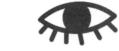

INTRODUCTION

Everyone is afraid of something. It could be dogs, public speaking, germs, or getting lost—the list is endless. Having some fear is a good thing. It's the reason we don't jump in front of moving cars or dive off tall buildings. Fear can literally keep us alive. The problems come when fear starts getting in the way of your life and keeps you from doing the things that are important to you. When that fear strikes, it often brings unwanted negative effects with it and impacts relationships, academic success, or future plans.

As a clinical psychologist, I've spent my career helping teens reverse these negative patterns using cognitive behavioral therapy (CBT) and mindfulness techniques. With practice, these skills can help you manage anxiety by changing your thoughts, behaviors, and physical reactions to better navigate life's challenges. We know these skills work, because they have been studied widely by researchers and used by therapists in many different settings. With this book, I hope to reach teens looking for ways to take back control of their lives.

This book will lay out practical exercises and techniques for coping with stress and anxiety. You can use a journal, notebook, or even the "Notes" app on your phone to record your progress and work on the exercises you want to try. You'll find exercises that fall under three categories:

+ **FOCUS:** Exercises like quizzes and assessments to help you better understand your anxiety

✳ **MINDFUL:** Practices designed to help you cope with your anxiety in the present moment

⚡ **ACTION:** Tools and exercises to develop skills to manage your anxiety in the long term

HOW TO USE THIS BOOK

Use this book in a way that's right for you. This book is a toolbox filled with a wide range of strategies and skills. Some skills will work better than others. Once you go through them and start practicing them regularly, you can figure out what works for you. Everyone will have their own starting point. Your goal is to integrate these skills into a consistent self-care plan that works for you.

If you don't know where to start, start small and simple. Begin with basic self-care like good sleep and regular exercise, or with an everyday awareness practice like tracking your moods. There will never be a perfect time to start. If you wait until you feel absolutely ready, you may never start. Waiting for that perfect time could be an avoidance or delay tactic—the very problem we're trying to address! That's why the perfect time to start is *now*, even if you only feel half ready.

Coping with anxiety is not one-size-fits-all, so decide what *you* want to change and use the exercises and skills to develop new habits. Your anxiety did not develop overnight, so it won't go away overnight either. But with practice, time, and dedication, you can begin to make little changes that can go a long way in making your life more enjoyable.

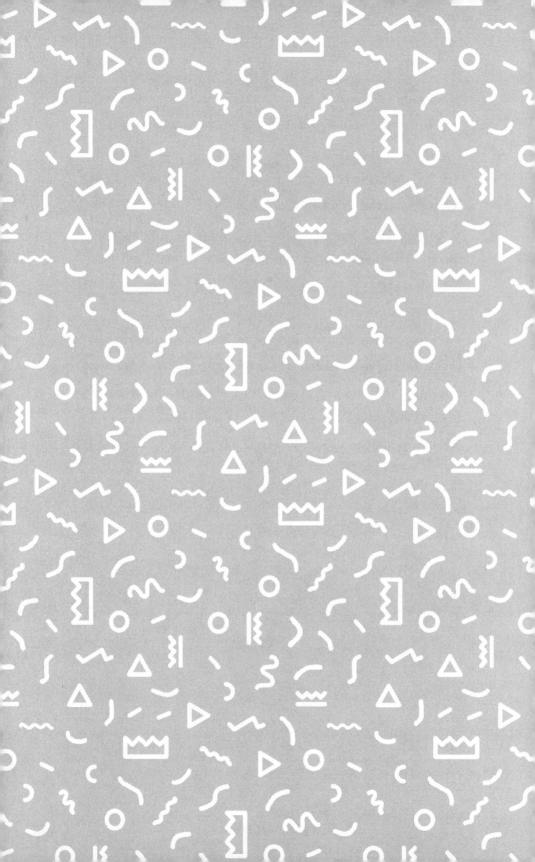

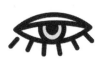

CHAPTER 1

YOU CAN RETRAIN YOUR BRAIN

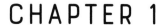

Teenagers juggle a ton of social, academic, and family responsibilities. Add stress and anxiety to the mix, and it's a wonder you get anything done! The fact that you're taking the time to read this is a pretty big first step—it means you're ready to make some changes. CBT and mindfulness will give you the skills you need to make those changes and be the person you want to be. But first, let's take a step back and look at what exactly it is you're wanting to change. Exploring this part of yourself may not be easy, but self-awareness is an important first step to positive change.

WHERE DOES ANXIETY COME FROM?

Anxiety is more common than you might think. It affects one in three teens, which means a good number of your classmates are dealing with similar problems. Researchers know that a mix of nature (your genetics) and nurture (your environment) influences how, when, and why anxiety shows up. Anxiety often runs in families, so that's a point for nature. Yet we also know that stressful life events like a big move, a parents' divorce, or a breakup can also play a big role.

Some anxiety is good for us. In fact, humans are hardwired to feel fear as a survival mechanism—it's our brain's natural reaction to dangerous situations. We even have a physical response to it called "fight, flight, or freeze." This response sets us up to defend ourselves, to escape, or to stop (think of a deer in headlights) when faced with an outside threat. It's an instinct that's kept our species alive for generations! But this same instinct can become a problem when the fight-flight-freeze response goes off too often, without any real danger triggers. Think of it like this: A caveman's fear of lions is good for his survival; your fear of talking to that cute new kid in class is probably not as helpful.

ANXIETY QUIZ

It's hard to handle a problem that feels nameless and faceless. This quiz can help you better understand the different types of anxiety. By naming the anxiety you feel, you can reach for specific tools and techniques to manage it. More often than not, anxiety comes in more than one form, so don't be surprised if more than one category applies to you, or if you chose all the statements in a specific category. That just means you're not alone in how you're feeling. I know there are a lot of statements here, so just be as honest as possible and mark any that may apply to you.

GENERALIZED ANXIETY

☐ I often get nervous about different things in my life like my health, academics, friendships, dating, or family.

☐ I worry about not being as good as my friends.

☐ I worry about whether things will work out for me in the future.

AGORAPHOBIA

☐ I stay home to avoid feeling uncomfortable or panicky.

☐ I need a specific person with me to face certain situations.

PHOBIAS

☐ I have a strong fear of something specific like:

    ☐ Blood or needles

    ☐ Dogs or other animals

    ☐ Storms and bad weather

    ☐ The dark

    ☐ High places or places where I feel enclosed

SOCIAL ANXIETY

☐ I get nervous around people I don't know well.

☐ It's hard for me to talk to people I don't know well.

☐ I am shy.

☐ I get nervous having to do something while other people watch me (reading aloud, public speaking, playing a sport).

☐ I feel nervous going to parties where I don't know people well.

SEPARATION ANXIETY

☐ I'm scared to sleep away from home, or worry about being away from my family.

☐ I prefer to stay close to my parents.

☐ I worry about something bad happening to my parents.

☐ I'm afraid to be alone at home or to sleep alone.

PANIC ATTACKS

☐ I often feel sick, even when nothing is actually medically wrong with me.

☐ I get frightened out of the blue.

☐ When I feel nervous:

    ☐ It's hard for me to breathe.

    ☐ I feel like passing out.

    ☐ I feel like I'll lose control.

    ☐ I feel like I'll go crazy.

    ☐ My heart beats fast.

    ☐ I get shaky.

    ☐ I sweat a lot.

    ☐ I feel like I'm choking.

    ☐ I feel dizzy.

OBSESSIVE-COMPULSIVE DISORDER (OCD)

☐ I'm bothered by obsessive thoughts I can't get rid of, like worries that I'm dirty or have germs on me, that someone else will get hurt because of something I did or didn't do, or that I'll do something shocking.

☐ I do things over and over that I can't resist doing, like counting, checking, washing, or straightening things up.

FORMS OF ANXIETY

Anxiety can take many different forms. Some are more physical, some are more related to mental worry, and some only manifest in specific situations. If you did the "Anxiety Quiz" (PAGE 7), the following defines these different types of anxiety.

GENERALIZED ANXIETY DISORDER is when you worry excessively about everyday things like home, school, or friends. These worries are difficult to control. You may expect the worst of situations or agonize more than others about things like an upcoming exam or a fight with a friend.

SOCIAL ANXIETY is a fear of being negatively judged or rejected by other people. You may worry about acting stupid or being boring, and this fear often leads you to avoid social interactions or situations where others might be watching.

SEPARATION ANXIETY is a fear of being away from people close to you, typically your parents. You might get anxious at just the thought of not being with them or imagine that the worst will happen while you're apart.

PHOBIAS are intense fears of specific situations, often to the point of being irrational because the fear does not match the reality of the threat. They typically focus on animals, insects, germs, extreme weather, or enclosed spaces. While it's normal to feel uncomfortable with these situations, most people can face them and go about their lives. With phobias, you may go out of your way to completely avoid these uncomfortable situations, even if you realize the fear is irrational.

PANIC ATTACKS are the physical manifestation of anxiety, where sudden, intense, and uncomfortable physical sensations make you feel like you're having a heart attack or going crazy. After having one panic attack, you may become fearful of having more, which is the hallmark of panic disorder. When fear of these panic attacks is so crippling that you stop going to school or leaving the house, or will only go to places with specific people, that's called **agoraphobia**.

OBSESSIVE-COMPULSIVE DISORDER, or OCD, involves thoughts that stick in your head and cause distress, for example, "That chair is teeming with germs!" The thoughts become so obsessive that you feel you must do *something*, say avoid the chair and wash your hands.

This behavior is called a compulsion. While compulsive behavior makes you feel better in the short term, it can actually lead to more obsessions that only make you more anxious, causing you to engage in even more compulsive behavior.

As you go through this book, you'll learn that different skills will be useful for different types of anxiety. For examples of how certain skills can be applied to various manifestations of anxiety, check out the Appendix (PAGE 168), where I've laid out some sample programs.

SO, WHAT ARE CBT AND MINDFULNESS?

Cognitive behavioral therapy, or CBT, is a set of skills designed to change the thoughts (the cognitive part) and actions (the behavior patterns) that get in the way of living a full and healthy life. The aim of CBT is to help you become your own therapist, and the skills are practical, goal-oriented, and can be practiced every day.

While some CBT strategies focus on changing thoughts or behaviors, others are rooted in mindfulness or awareness- and acceptance-based approaches. You may have noticed that when you're anxious about something, your thoughts are everywhere but *here*—you fret about the past, or about how things could go wrong in the future. Mindfulness helps focus your attention on whatever you're doing right *now*, in the present moment.

Acceptance strategies help you cope with, and even accept, uncomfortable situations or emotions that you can't control or change.

While this may seem counterintuitive, since the anxiety you're experiencing is exactly what you're trying to escape, it's actually that desire to escape the present moment that often causes anguish. Focusing your full attention on the present and accepting your discomfort can help you realize that the thing you're trying to get away from is not as overwhelming as you thought it would be.

CBT WORKS

CBT is shown to work for all types of anxiety, but these skills can also be helpful for other negative emotions such as depression and anger. We also know it can help improve sleep, reduce chronic pain, help people with eating disorders and with addiction, and help people manage tics and skin picking.

In my practice, the goal is to build a toolbox. When you have a comprehensive toolbox, you can fix most problems. Hanging a picture? Grab a hammer. Building furniture? Get the drill. The right CBT and mindfulness tools can apply to most parts of your life, and once you start using them, you can start feeling, thinking, and acting like the person you want to be.

One thing that amazes me is how quickly CBT works. A high school sophomore came in recently complaining that her stomach was constantly upset. She had been to multiple doctors who had ruled out any physical illness. We quickly pinpointed how her worry about getting nauseous was making her even more nauseous, and how she was avoiding places where she might start thinking about her stomach problems. We put a plan in place where she began to face her fears by going places where she felt nauseous, and she used coping skills to manage her anxiety when she felt it coming on. She went from having these symptoms once a day to once a month, and told me that they were way more manageable than she would have expected. She was confident in her new skills and sure that she could handle the symptoms when they did crop up.

ANXIETY IS ADAPTIVE

Picture this: You're Kronk the Caveman. You hear a rustling noise behind you and think, "Oh, that's probably just Grog, back from his berry picking." You don't even look up from your pile of sticks as you say, "Hey Grog, it's your turn to patrol the cave." But it turns out it's not Grog, it's a tiger, and it pounces before you have a chance to process. Not a very good day for Kronk.

Now, scenario B: You hear a rustling noise behind you, and your hair automatically stands on end. Your heart beats faster, you start to sweat, and your muscles tense up. You scan the perimeter of your cave and notice movement in the bushes. You think, "This must be dangerous!" and run into your safe cave, evading the tiger and surviving another day.

A fear response to actual danger is adaptive, healthy, and lifesaving. But responding with anxiety to situations that are not actually dangerous can get in the way of your functioning. Think of a smoke alarm: When there's a fire, the smoke alarm provides an important signal to leave the house or put out a fire. When the smoke alarm goes off without an actual fire, it's a nuisance. Imagine if every time a false alarm sounded, you responded as if there were a real fire by grabbing the fire extinguisher, running out of the house, and calling 911—all because you burned a slice of bread in the toaster! Anxiety is a false alarm that signals danger even when it isn't present. Our goal is to learn strategies to treat these experiences like false alarms rather than true fires.

THE CBT MODEL OF EMOTIONS

CBT breaks emotions down into three parts: thoughts, physical sensations, and behaviors. Say you're afraid of dogs and you see a dog coming toward you along the sidewalk. You feel afraid—that's your emotion. You think, "That dog might bite me!"—that's the thought. Your palms get sweaty, your breath quickens, and your heart speeds up—that's the physical sensation. And finally, you cross to the other side of the street—that's your behavior. As you can see, your emotions, thoughts, sensations, and behaviors are interconnected, and each of these parts plays a role in maintaining and strengthening the emotion that you feel. Each of these parts can trigger a full-blown anxiety cycle.

It's important to note that there's always a trigger to anxiety— it may just be hard to identify because our reactions are often so

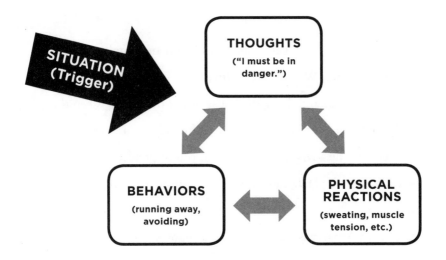

automatic. Changing one of these parts—thoughts, sensations, or behaviors—can help you break out of the cycle. For example, if you were in the same exact situation but thought, "Hey, that's a really adorable dog," you probably wouldn't cross the street or notice those bodily sensations. Or if you had kept walking without avoiding the dog, you might have learned that it was harmless, which might in turn lead to less anxiety the next time you face a dog.

You might be wondering why you've never noticed these separate but interconnected factors before. When you're in the thick of a negative emotion, everything is just an overwhelming blur of fear and anxiety. Our goal is to help you break down these anxiety tornados so you can tease out the pieces and manage them separately instead of getting lost in them.

Here's another way to show how connected these pieces are: If you start feeling sweaty and notice your breathing speed up, you might think, "Whoa, something is wrong with my body." If you think something is wrong, your heart might start racing or your muscles might tense up. That unpleasant bodily response just confirms that something really *is* wrong with your body, so you try to do something to get rid of the sensations, like running to the kitchen to drink a glass of water. This behavior seems like a great move, but since you are feeling nervous, you drop the glass on the floor and spill water everywhere—which only makes you more anxious! You can see how this creates an endless cycle of anxiety in the diagram below:

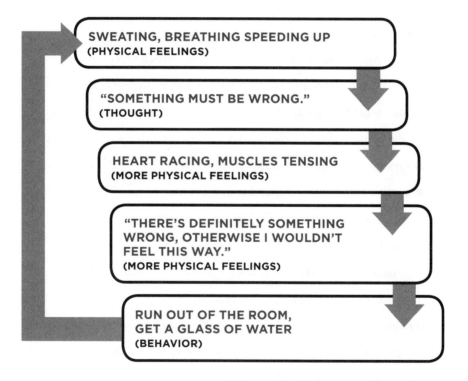

If you had stayed in the situation and observed how your sensations affected your thoughts and behavior, you might have noticed that in most situations, even the most unpleasant thoughts and sensations gradually go away on their own. Anxiety tries to get you to escape or avoid unpleasant situations. That may provide short-term relief, but it doesn't show you how to handle the situation the next time it comes up, which it probably will.

HOW AVOIDANCE KEEPS ANXIETY GOING

Let's say you have a paper due next week. You aren't sure where to start, which makes you feel anxious. You may think, "I'll never get this done in time." You may also notice some changes in your body—your hands start to get sweaty, your muscles feel tight, and your stomach starts to turn. That's a subtle fight-flight-freeze response, your body's way of telling you you're anxious. So you blow off the paper and spend the night FaceTiming with friends. You can always start tomorrow instead, right? You feel great until tomorrow, when you still have the paper due but less time to do it! In the short term, avoidance makes you feel better. In the long term, it leaves you with fewer skills and feeling worse.

Avoidance can also spiral really quickly. Although it's the quickest way to feel better, it can actually cause *more* unpleasant thoughts and sensations over time. If you need to give an oral presentation to your class and it makes you feel anxious, you can run out of the room and avoid that specific presentation. But what are you going to do next time? And the time after that? And what if your classmates now think of you as the girl who runs out of the room when she's called on? In this scenario, you've let anxiety get in the way of your long-term growth as a student. In Chapter 5, we'll discuss more about avoidance and beneficial skills to use instead.

UNCOVERING YOUR TRIGGERS

Anxiety always has a trigger. A good way to identify your triggers is to ask yourself a simple question: What happened before you felt anxious? Triggers don't have to be specific events (though they can be). They can also be thoughts or physical sensations, or even behaviors. Any part of the anxiety cycle can start the spiral.

The good news is that changing any part of the cycle can keep your anxiety from spiraling out of control. We're often so caught up in how bad anxiety feels that we have trouble noticing when and how it starts. Like a scientist collecting data, being able to just notice what you're thinking or feeling in the moment can give you important clues about what skills to use. I call this building awareness, or mindfulness.

Know that triggers can be internal or external. An external trigger is anything that happens outside your body or self, like a fight with a friend, an exam, or a doctor's appointment. An internal trigger can be a personal belief or thought or a bodily sensation. If you're not sure what triggers your anxiety, you can use the exercises in "Track Your Anxiety" (PAGE 23) to begin figuring it out.

EXTRA SUPPORT

This book is here to show you how to help yourself, but sometimes anxiety can be a lot to handle alone. If your anxiety feels overwhelming, talk to an adult you can trust, like a parent, a teacher, or a counselor. Here are some signs that you may need extra help:

- Do you think about hurting yourself?

- Do you ever wish you were dead?

- Are you feeling hopeless?

- Do you drink alcohol or smoke to numb or escape your feelings?

- Have you thought about killing yourself?

If you wish you were dead or have thoughts about hurting yourself, that's a signal that you need to talk to someone right away. You can text "HOME" to 741741 or call **1-800-273-TALK (8255)** 24 hours a day, seven days a week, for support. If you'd like to find a therapist, especially one who practices the CBT or mindfulness skills outlined in this book, you can check out the websites listed in the references section on PAGE 173.

STAYING ON TRACK

The skills and strategies in this book are meant to be put into practice, not just read. Practicing new skills is like wearing new shoes—they might pinch a little when you first try them on, and you might not be sure if you're going to like walking around in them. It could take a couple wears to break them in enough that they feel truly yours. To break in your skills and get the most out of this book, follow some of these tips:

- **Don't be afraid to ask for support.** Think about the people in your life who make you feel safe and let them know what you're doing. If it's helpful to have someone stay on top of you, ask a supportive person to check in with you every now and then. If you learn by talking things out, find someone who will listen.

- **Just because you need something right now doesn't mean you'll always need it.** Your needs might change as you progress. If you ask a parent for help with skills but they end up driving you crazy by constantly checking up on you, you can ask them to leave you alone or give you more space. That's OK. This is about what works for *you*.

- **The best way to climb a ladder is one rung at a time.** Celebrate the small steps and achievements—they're the things that get you to the big steps.

- **Be open to learning new skills.** Some of these tools might feel weird or nerdy, but they're proven to work. Just give them a try! You can always start somewhere safe where no one's watching, like your bedroom.

- **Know when to practice (and when not to!).** Don't try a strategy for the first time when you're in freak-out mode—it'll be hard for new information to stick if you're in an anxiety spiral. A good time to try some of these skills, like journaling or mood tracking, is before bed while you unwind.

- **Be kind to yourself.** If you get off track because life gets busy, just return to the exercises and skills whenever you can and pick up where you left off.

- **Keep practicing!** Preferably on a daily basis. It's normal for a skill to not "work" the first time around. You would never try to compete at the Olympics after your first cartwheel!

TRACK YOUR ANXIETY

Self-awareness is something we will work on throughout this book, since it is the foundation for managing difficult emotions and thoughts. One important way to manage anxiety is to start observing when and how it is triggered. Here's how:

1. **Start keeping a running list.** Make note of when you feel anxious, and what happened right before or during. It doesn't have to be complicated—list the day, time, and what was going on. For example, you can write: "Tuesday, play rehearsal, heart racing."

2. **Pick a time of day to do your tracking.** If you're worried that you'll be making notes all day long, you can do this or track consistently for a day or two to give yourself a feel for "a day in the life."

3. **You can write in code or shorthand.** This is helpful if you worry about other people seeing what you're writing. You can fill it in for yourself later when you're in private.

4. **Look for patterns.** Writing things down will let you see patterns like times of day, events, or people involved, all details that help you identify triggers. If you notice that you're always anxious right before lunch, then boom—we found a trigger.

5. **Try to begin ranking how anxious you are on a scale of 0 to 10.** Ten is the most anxious you've ever been; 0 is the calmest. Just be aware that 10 is the ceiling—there's nothing higher than that. If you tell me you're afraid of heights, and that standing on the second floor of school was a 10, I'm going to ask, "OK, well what about the fifth floor? Is that the same?" If the answer is "No, that's a higher ten," then maybe the second floor was more like an 8. This is not an exact science, but it'll give you a sense of how you experience anxiety in different situations.

MONITOR YOUR THOUGHTS, FEELINGS, AND BEHAVIORS

Start breaking down those emotions! This is a helpful way to begin understanding how you experience those three parts of the CBT model of anxiety. To begin, pick an event that happened recently that made you feel anxious. Ask yourself the following questions:

- **What was I thinking when that situation happened?**
- **What was my physical reaction?**
- **What did I do?**

These questions seem easy, but don't be surprised if this is harder than you thought. It's a new way of thinking about anxiety, so it's common to struggle with pinpointing what you were thinking or feeling in any given moment or situation. It might be helpful to map things out as follows:

- **Situation:** I got anxious in math class on Wednesday when the teacher assigned hard homework.
- **Thoughts:** "I won't be able to get any of it right and I'll fail, or my friends will think I'm stupid if I ask them for help."

- **Physical sensation:** My muscles tensed up.
- **Behavior:** I procrastinated until the last minute and then rushed to finish.

Getting in the habit of thinking about your triggers, thoughts, physical sensations, and behaviors will help you be more aware of them. More awareness equals more opportunity to make a dent in that anxiety. This is a good exercise to do once a week or so. Over time, you'll notice it gets easier to break down your emotions and experiences in this way.

SHORT- AND LONG-TERM CONSEQUENCES

Once you're tracking your thoughts, sensations, and behaviors, you can start reflecting on why you act the way you do. Let's take the example of procrastinating on math homework.

- **What are the short-term benefits of this behavior?** Pushing off my math homework means I don't have to do it right now, which is great for me in the moment. I can watch Netflix all night!
- **On the other hand, what are the long-term consequences of procrastination?** Well, since I pushed it off till the last minute, I had to rush to finish my homework. I made more errors than I would have with more time, which only reinforced my belief that I wouldn't be able to get any of it right. I didn't get the practice I needed to do well in math.

What if I reversed the example and buckled down and did my math homework even though I felt anxious about it? Then the consequences would be switched around.

- **Short-term consequences:** I'm stressed out all night and worry that I'm doing the homework all wrong. I keep having to erase and double-check my answers.
- **Long-term consequences:** I turned my homework in on time and actually made fewer mistakes than if I'd rushed. I feel really proud of myself for pushing through the anxiety and getting it done!

Sometimes we get so stuck in anxiety that it feels like quicksand. We try desperately to escape it and just end up getting even more stuck. By trying to avoid difficulties, we often create situations that only lead to more distress—that's how we get caught up in anxiety spirals! Taking time to think about the immediate and long-term consequences of avoidant behavior can help you recognize when and how your anxiety causes problems. In this way, you can come up with a plan for getting yourself unstuck.

VISUALIZE THE NEW YOU

What would your life look like if there was a magic button that you could press and make your anxiety disappear? Visualization is a way to imagine how you might be different if you approached life's challenges differently. Find a comfortable spot and take 15 minutes of your day to do the following:

1. **Imagine yourself without anxiety.** What changes might other people notice in your mood or demeanor? Would you stop avoiding the cafeteria? Could you be in a room with a spider without freaking out? How would your relationships be different? Study habits? Social and extracurricular activities? Be as specific as you can by putting yourself in past or future situations.

2. **In a journal or notebook, write down this different version of yourself.**

3. **Now think about your motivation.** Take a few minutes to reflect on *why* you want to change.

4. **Write these reasons down in your journal.** You can always revisit this list if things get tough and you feel you need a reminder.

5. **Now think about the things that are getting in the way of making positive changes.** Maybe you don't know where to start (reading this book is a good place!), maybe it seems too hard, or maybe it's the time commitment.

6. **Write these obstacles down in your journal.** If you're honest with yourself about what's getting in the way, you can begin applying problem-solving skills to those roadblocks. This is the only way to move closer to the new version of yourself that you've visualized.

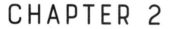

CHAPTER 2

THE MIND-BODY CONNECTION

It's impossible to talk about your mind without talking about your body. After all, your brain is literally *inside* your body! We know anxiety has a physical component—it can make your muscles tense or your palms sweaty, for example. And we know that physical health impacts mental well-being, like when having a cold makes you grumpy or sad. A core approach to overcoming anxiety is becoming more aware of how your bodily sensations impact your thoughts and emotions, and vice versa, so you are better able to manage them all as they arise.

TAKING CARE OF YOUR BODY

What do you do to keep your body healthy? Sleep, exercise, nutrition, and stress can all affect your mood for better or worse. When you're feeling down and stay in bed all day, do you feel better or do you just feel worse for doing nothing all day? When you stay up all night stressing out about school, how does that impact your ability to function? Are you irritable and unable to focus in class the next day? How we take care of our body says a lot about how we take care of our mind.

Some people use the words "stress" and "anxiety" interchangeably, but they're actually two different things. Stress is what you feel when faced with external pressures that you can't control but are a normal part of life. Life stressors can include a fight between your parents, an upcoming final, a big sports tournament, or a friend's birthday party. Anxiety, on the other hand, is an emotion that you might feel *in response* to stress. In other words, it's a reflection of how well you're able to cope with life's stressors. Being aware of this distinction is key to keeping stress from turning into anxiety. Since the mind and body are connected, taking good care of your body will help you be more mentally prepared to handle the stresses that come your way, so you can be healthier, happier, and less anxious.

A PROPER NIGHT'S SLEEP

Even though it can be tough, you should make it a priority to get enough sleep. Sleep is like eating: Too much or too little can impact how you feel. Research shows that people who get enough sleep do better on exams, and have improved memory and mood, compared to those who don't. People with insomnia (chronic problems falling or staying asleep) are much more likely to experience anxiety or depression. It can be hard to detect how a few nights of poor sleep impact your mood, but even a little bit of sleep deprivation can throw you off your game and heighten your anxiety levels. Quality of sleep impacts quality of life because it regulates eating and metabolism and helps us better manage stress.

You might notice that you started staying up later once you hit high school. There's a biological reason for that—our sleep rhythms shift as we age, so you naturally stay awake later. But you still need to get up early for school, and experts recommend that teens get 8 to 10 hours of sleep a night to function well and feel healthy. This is the range for an "average" teen, but everyone is different. To figure out how much sleep your body needs, consider the following:

- **How long do you sleep when you feel well rested, say during vacation or on weekends when you've recovered from late study nights, camp, or other activities?**
- **In your journal, write down the time you go to bed on these nights when you feel well rested. Do this a few days in a row.**
- **For these same days of good sleep, write down the time you naturally wake up without an alarm.**
- **Figure out the average number of hours you slept on those nights. This number is a good guideline for how many hours of sleep your body naturally needs each night.**

ARE YOU GETTING ENOUGH SLEEP?

Getting good sleep is about having good sleeping habits, or what we call "sleep hygiene." To begin developing better habits, it's good to have a sense of how well you are sleeping right now. Here are some ways to know whether you're getting enough sleep:

1. Do you fall asleep within 15 minutes (give or take) of hitting the pillow?
2. Do you get between 8 and 10 hours of sleep a night?
3. Do you wake up before your alarm goes off?
4. Do you wake up in the middle of the night and have trouble going back to sleep?
5. Do you find yourself falling asleep or nodding off during the day?

If you answered yes to questions 1, 2, and 3, chances are you're getting a proper night's sleep. If you answered no to those questions, and yes to questions 4 and 5, then you're having some difficulty getting proper sleep. Check "Fall Asleep Faster" (PAGE 35) for some tips on improving your sleep.

FALL ASLEEP FASTER

Want to get to sleep faster and have better-quality sleep? Looking to your own sleep habits and behavior (both during the day and at bedtime) is a good starting point. These simple and effective sleep tips can make a difference:

- **Have a sleep schedule, even on weekends.** Pick a bedtime and a wake-up time, and stick to them. Life will interfere, but do the best you can. The goal is to consistently get the amount of sleep you need.

- **Use the "no glow rule."** Turn off electronic screens at least 30 minutes before your set bedtime. Phones and TVs emit blue light, which suppresses melatonin, the hormone your brain produces to fall asleep. Blue-light screens basically trick your brain into thinking it's still daytime! If your device has a blue light filter, turn it on an hour before bed.

- **Make bedtime a technology-free zone.** Devices can harm your sleep by just being next to you. Those late-night beeps and notifications keep your brain alert instead of giving it a chance to unwind. If you have to use your phone as an alarm clock, try putting it in a box once you're ready to sleep so you don't see it.

- **Create a relaxing bedtime ritual.** Read a book, write in your journal, or listen to music. Do a meditation like the ones in this chapter. Bedtime is a perfect time to incorporate mindfulness practices or progressive muscle relaxation into your schedule.

- **Make your bedroom a good environment for sleep.** Create a space that allows you to relax and fall asleep with ease. Make sure the temperature is comfortable and turn the lights off. Even the alarm clock light can affect sleep, so turn it around if you find that it keeps you up.

- **Exercise regularly. (But not after 9 p.m.!)** To state the obvious, exercise helps tire your body out. Just don't do any push-ups at bedtime—the adrenaline will keep you up!

- **Avoid caffeine, especially after lunch.** The stimulant effects of caffeine stay in your system for hours and can affect the quality of your sleep. So put down the soda at dinnertime and drink some water instead.

It's normal to stay up late every now and then. But if you have insomnia, there's a specific CBT program that can help you, called CBT for Insomnia, or CBT-I. Check out the Resources section for more details.

MOVE YOUR BODY

We've known for a while that moving your body is good for your physical health, and now more and more research shows a positive connection between movement and mental health. Thirty minutes of exercise five days a week can reduce feelings of depression, increase positive emotions, and help you manage stress throughout the day. And as exercise even helps you sleep better!

If you already do sports, dance, or go to the gym, great! If not, here are some ways to build physical activity into your day:

- **Start small.** Ten minutes is better than nothing, and all movement counts. You might already be moving more than you think! Take the stairs instead of the elevator, or get off the bus one stop early and walk home. (Bonus points if your backpack adds a little weight!)

- **Find something active that you enjoy.** If you hate running, don't force yourself to join the track team—you'll just be setting yourself up for disappointment. Instead, think about ways to move that appeal to you. It could be playing a dancing video game after school, taking a bike ride, or walking your dog.

- **Find a friend.** Exercising with a buddy is a good way to build accountability (in other words, forcing yourself to actually do it), and can also make it more enjoyable.

- **Download an app.** There are many great phone apps that will take the guesswork out of what to do and how. For example, the Couch to 5k app helps you get into a running routine, and the 7-Minute Workout app offers options for quick, high-intensity sweat sessions.

With exercise especially, small steps are better than nothing, and little steps can have a big impact. Think small and doable, and build on those small steps when you're ready.

STAYING IN THE PRESENT WITH MINDFULNESS

Think about all the time you spend worrying about the future or the past. It's common to make contingency plans for possible future disasters or to replay things that went wrong over and over in our minds. But isn't it incredibly draining? Mindfulness involves a completely different way of living life. It helps us ground in the present moment so we don't get so caught up in that negative cycle of worries and plans.

Mindfulness means paying full attention to your experience on a moment-to-moment basis. When you practice mindfulness, you can notice what's happening and accept it for what it is, rather than obsessing over what you wish it could be. Often, anxiety is all about being "in your head." If you're always judging your experience and thoughts, then you're letting those reactive feelings control you. If you're anxious about what a friend thinks of you, you may focus on the details of your most recent interaction (the past), or worry about what will happen the next time you see them (the future). By focusing your attention on whatever is happening right now, you can begin to let go of those other anxieties and learn to better manage your emotions as they arise.

Note that this is different from relaxation techniques. The goal of mindfulness is not necessarily to relax; it's to be in full awareness of what's happening right now—be it thoughts, emotions, sensations, actions, or events. Sometimes that can help you relax, but sometimes it won't. Instead, mindfulness helps you accept, notice, and tolerate your emotions and the situations that you find yourself in. The research on mindfulness shows that it is linked to positive benefits in areas like:

- **Improving attention span**
- **Improving mood, including decreased anxiety and depression in adults**
- **Regulating emotions**
- **Reacting less strongly and more flexibly to challenges**
- **Building happier relationships**
- **Showing more compassion toward other people**
- **Accepting more compassion from other people**

MINDFULNESS, THE BASICS

Mindfulness is awareness of the present moment without judgment. It reduces suffering by taking you out of the worry and rumination that feed anxiety. Psychologists teach mindfulness practice through visualization, breathing, meditation, and other exercises. It's a skill that you build over time, like strengthening a muscle. Focusing your attention fully on the present can be hard, because it means returning to what you're doing over and over, even when you get distracted. You might worry that you aren't very good at it (and that thought itself is a distraction!). It's normal to feel this way, so that's why the best way to develop mindfulness skills in everyday life is to practice in brief sessions. One minute a day, consistently, can be enough to start off.

Learning and understanding how these skills work can be tough. I was working with a teen with migraines and anxiety and realized mindfulness could be a really helpful tool for him. When I introduced mindfulness meditation, he dismissed it as "dumb breathing" and almost dropped out of therapy. A few months later, when we were reviewing his progress, I asked him what skill he found most helpful when he was in pain, and he sheepishly responded that the breathing made a huge difference. I didn't say "I told you so," but I was totally thinking it. Mindfulness helped him accept the pain and recognize that he could handle it. By giving the headache some attention in a nonjudgmental way, he was able to release tension and move past it.

The mindfulness exercises in this book are designed to help you focus your attention on the here and now. Try them out, and use the ones that work for you. *Your main job is to observe what you're doing without getting involved.* Here are some basic rules to keep in mind while you practice:

- **Imagine yourself as a drone.** You can see everything that's going on, but you're detached from it because you're a machine.
- **Don't focus on the outcome.** Your only job is to observe what's going on in an objective way.
- **While you're observing, try describing what you see or feel to yourself.**
- **As you describe, remember to hold off on judgment.** It's not about bad or good, or right or wrong; it's about taking it all in.
- **You will get distracted, because you're human and that's how our minds work.** When you do, return your attention to whatever you were noticing in a gentle, nonjudgmental way. If you catch yourself judging or thinking things like "This isn't even helping" or "I must be doing this wrong," try being kind and compassionate to yourself. It's OK if this all seems too philosophical or unclear at first. That's why the most important part is the *practice.*

PREPARING FOR MINDFUL PRACTICE

If you play a sport, what do you do to learn and perfect a new skill? One word: practice. Athletes stick to specific exercise regimens designed to get them into shape. Mindfulness is like a muscle, so treat it like you would a sport. Would you expect to be in better shape after doing one jumping jack? Of course not! Approaching mindfulness this way will help you combat any obstacles or excuses down the line.

- **MAKE A SCHEDULE.** How many days a week will you practice? At what time? The more specific you can be, the better. This will help get rid of excuses like "I didn't have time!"

- **CREATE A SPACE AND TIME TO PRACTICE.** This could be while you're lying in bed before falling asleep or on your way to or from school.

- **PICK AN EXERCISE TO TRY REPEATEDLY.** It can be any of the mindfulness exercises in this book. Try an exercise for at least a week. Remember, if mindfulness is like exercise, doing something once is not enough to learn.

- **CONSISTENCY MATTERS.** Thirty seconds of breathing meditation every single day is better than a longer exercise only when you happen to remember. To start, choose something simple and short enough that you can do it every day, even at your worst (and if you forget, that's OK too, just get back to it tomorrow).

- **KEEP TRACK!** Set up a simple chart with a box for each day of the week. Check off when you've done your daily mindfulness activity, and note which activity you completed. Ask yourself if you feel better, worse, or the same after the activity. For some people, checking that box can be great motivation to keep going. If writing things down doesn't work for you, that's OK—just try to find a way to practice mindfulness every day.

- **STAY OPEN.** Keep your mind open to experiencing and noticing what mindfulness practice feels like, and stay curious as you try out these new skills.

DO ONE THING AT A TIME

USEFUL FOR: Building mindfulness into your day
by focusing on what you're doing right now

TIME: Varies, but daily

When was the last time you focused completely on a single task or activity? If you're like most people, you probably try to do many things at once. You might study while eating, check e-mail while watching TV, or plan your day in the shower. Multitasking is totally normal, but it also means you're never fully present for one thing. Focusing and doing one thing at a time is a great way to begin incorporating mindfulness into your day, especially if you don't always have time for a formal practice!

1. **Pick an activity you do every day, like brushing your teeth, taking a shower, or packing your lunch.**
2. **As you complete this task, try to be fully in the moment.** Use as many senses as you can to keep your attention on that task and nothing else.

For example, if you're showering:

- Notice how the water feels as it comes into contact with your skin.
- Pay attention to the temperature.
- When you pick up the soap, notice how it feels in your hand and as you're washing.
- What does the water look like? What does the soap smell like?
- If your thoughts wander, bring them back to the experience of taking a shower.

3. **After you try this one activity for a week, take note of any changes in yourself or in the experience.** And if you don't notice any changes at first, that's OK!

TIP:

Remember that it's normal to get distracted. If you lose focus, just bring your attention back to what you're doing, without judgment.

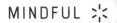
LAKE MEDITATION

USEFUL FOR: Stress relief; connecting with your calm self

TIME: 10 minutes

Mindfulness meditation can help relieve anxiety by connecting with a steady, calm part of yourself. This exercise is good for when you feel like situations are chaotic or out of control and you need to return to a calmer place.

1. **Lie down in a comfortable position and close your eyes.**
2. **Bring awareness to your body.** Notice the sensations as you settle in. Notice the points of contact between your body and the surface on which you are lying.
3. **Once you're comfortable, imagine a lake.** It can be a lake you've visited or one you've seen in pictures. Visualize it. Is it big or small? Is it perfectly round or oddly shaped? Take in the scenery. Is it surrounded by trees? Are there mountains?
4. **Bring your attention to the lake's surface.** Notice how it changes depending on the time of day. The color may change depending on the light, or darken when clouds block the sun. Beneath the surface, though, the water stays the same throughout the day.

5. **Notice also how the lake's surface changes with the weather.** When rain beats down, the water may churn. When the wind blows, it may ripple with waves. With a change of seasons, the lake's surface might freeze into ice in the winter, or be covered with dried leaves in the fall. It might warm up under the heat of the summer sun. With all these changes, though, the bottom of the lake remains still and undisturbed.

6. **The lake's surface is the world you live in.** It will change with time and external factors that might be out of your control. But these changes don't have to affect your sense of well-being. As you meditate, focus on becoming the entirety of the lake. Observe the thoughts, sensations, and situations that disturb the surface, while also connecting with the stillness that is always somewhere inside of you. The stillness is as much a part of the lake as the waves and ripples. Let yourself feel the calmness of these deep waters, and know that you can return to it when you feel overwhelmed by what's happening on the surface of your lake.

TIP:

Find a consistent time to build this exercise (or another meditation if this one doesn't work for you) into your schedule. Lying in bed is a good time for many teens, because it can help you clear your mind and relax before falling asleep.

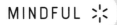
MINDFUL EATING

USEFUL FOR: Everyday mindfulness

TIME: 5 minutes

This eating exercise can give you a sense of how to incorporate mindfulness into your everyday life. Observe how eating this way—slowly, mindfully—is different from how you normally eat this food. You may notice how your eating experience changes when you slow down and focus your attention.

1. **Choose a small piece of food.** For example, you can choose a raisin, a single M&M, or a Hershey's Kiss. In this activity, you are a scientist, and your aim is to examine the food with all your senses as if discovering it for the first time.

2. **Hold the item in your palm and look closely at it.** What do you notice visually? Observe details—like the color and shape of the food. Describe it to yourself as a scientist would.

3. **What does it feel like?** Is the texture smooth? Rough? Hot? Cold? Smooth? Sticky? Observe the sensation in your hand.

4. **If the item has a wrapper, unwrap it.** Notice the texture of the wrapper and any changes in what you are now looking at.

5. **Use your sense of smell.** What does it smell like when you hold it up to your nose?

6. **Does the food make any sounds?** Hold it up to your ear and shake or squeeze it gently. Do you hear anything? Describe that to yourself.

7. **Put the item in your mouth—but don't chew it yet!** Let it rest on your tongue and notice what it feels like. What do you taste? Are there any new sensations in your mouth?

8. **Start slowly chewing.** Take one bite at a time. How do the taste and texture change in your mouth as you chew?

9. **Swallow the food.** As you swallow, how does the food feel going down your throat? Observe any sensations and describe them to yourself.

PROGRESSIVE MUSCLE RELAXATION

USEFUL FOR: Everyday stress relief and relaxation; releasing tension in your body

TIME: 10 minutes, once a day

Anxiety often shows up as physical strain and tight muscles. By tensing and then relaxing each muscle group, this exercise can help you become more aware of bodily sensations and feel more physically at ease. You'll be tensing each muscle group for 5 to 10 seconds. Don't completely tighten your muscles, since that can hurt. Instead, aim for about 75 percent muscle tension, then release the tension and relax the muscle for about 15 seconds. Notice the difference between tension and relaxation.

1. **Sit down comfortably and bring your attention to your breathing.**
2. **Squeeze your right hand and arm.** Hold for 10 to 15 seconds and then relax, letting go of any tension. Do the same with your left hand and arm. Repeat this cycle one more time.
3. **Turn your attention to your arms and shoulders.** Stretch your arms up into the air and back. Feel the pull in your shoul-

ders as you tense and hold. Now drop your arms to the side and relax for 15 seconds. Repeat.

4. **Focus on your shoulders and neck.** Pull your shoulders up toward your ears and feel the tension. Relax, drop your shoulders, and feel the difference between tension and relaxation before doing it once more.

5. **Turn your attention to your jaw.** Tense by biting down, and feel the tension in your jaw and neck muscles. Relax and let your jaw hang freely before repeating.

6. **Tense your face.** Scrunch your nose and forehead together and squeeze your eyes closed. (If this feels a little silly, just do it when nobody's watching!) Hold and relax before repeating. Notice if your face feels more relaxed.

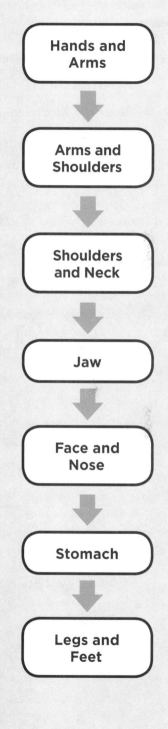

7. **Focus your attention on your stomach**. Squeeze in your abdomen, pulling your muscles toward your spine. Now let that tension go and feel your belly relax and expand. Repeat once.

8. **Tense the muscles in your right leg and foot.** Raise your leg and flex your toes toward the ceiling. Relax and let your foot rest on the floor again. Repeat with the left side, relax for 15 seconds, and cycle through once more.

TIP:

It may be useful to record yourself reading the steps and then play it back and follow along, and even close your eyes if that helps you focus (just try not to fall asleep!). With regular practice you might begin noticing tension in your body more automatically, and you can focus on relaxing specific muscles rather than doing the complete exercise.

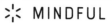

FIVE SENSES ACTIVITY, OR 5-4-3-2-1

USEFUL FOR: Grounding yourself quickly

TIME: 1 minute

Mindfulness can help you cope with internal anxiety by focusing attention on the external environment instead. This is useful when your thoughts and emotions feel chaotic and out of control. Grounding exercises like this one can take you out of your head and back into the present moment. It doesn't require a quiet place or a lot of time, just a shift in your attention.

1. **Look around you and name five things you can see.** Try to identify things you would not normally notice.
2. **Name four things you can touch.** Bring your focus to those items or surfaces as you feel them with your hand or body.
3. **Name three things you can hear from where you are.** It can be the ticking of a clock, the hum of an appliance, or a car passing by. Try to notice sounds you would normally ignore.
4. **Name two things you can smell.** These smells can be pleasant or unpleasant. Try noticing them without judgment.

5. **Name one thing you can taste**. If there's nothing within reach, do you notice any tastes or sensations in your mouth? If that's too challenging, name one flavor you like to taste instead.

TIP:

If you finish this exercise and are still overwhelmed by thoughts or emotions, you can do it again until the strong feelings pass.

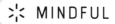

COLOR BREATHING

USEFUL FOR: Everyday relaxation; promoting calm

TIME: 5 minutes

Breathing exercises can help manage stress, regulate emotions, and even reduce blood pressure. This one combines abdominal breathing with visualization to help you clear your mind.

1. **Choose two colors:** one that you associate with relaxation, and another that you associate with anxiety or just don't like. For me, blue is calming, while yellow reminds me of caution tape. I'll use them in this example, but you can choose whatever colors work for you.

2. **Find a quiet place.** Sit or lie down in a comfortable position. Close your eyes and begin to focus on your breathing.

3. **Breathe in.** Imagine the color blue filling your lungs. Picture the color washing over your body with a sense of calm. Breathe the blue into all the parts of your body that feel extra tense.

4. **Exhale.** Visualize yourself breathing out the color yellow. That tense and anxious air is sticky and holds on tight inside your body, so the best way to release it is with long and slow breaths.

5. **Continue to visualize.** See the blue air filling your body with a sense of calm as you inhale and the yellow air leaving your body as you exhale. Feel your breath lengthen as you continue this exercise, and try to make your exhales longer than your inhales.

TIP:
This exercise is a good one to incorporate into your bedtime routine to clear your mind before falling asleep.

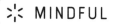

BODY SCAN

USEFUL FOR: Noticing and managing
physical symptoms of anxiety

TIME: 10 minutes

Since anxiety often shows up in our bodies, noticing physical sensations as they arise can be a huge help in managing stress before it snowballs. This exercise is one way of bringing greater awareness to physical sensations. If you experience a lot of physical symptoms of anxiety, it can be hard to focus on them at first, but the long-term benefits are worth it. It helps to record yourself reading the instructions out loud. You can then play it back and follow along.

1. **Sit upright in a chair with your feet flat on the floor, or lie on your back if you prefer.** Once you're comfortable, notice how your body feels sitting or lying down, paying attention to where it makes contact with the surfaces you are touching.
2. **Close your eyes and bring awareness to your breath.** Take a few long, deep breaths. Notice how each inhale feels as your breath fills your body and how each exhale feels as the breath leaves your body.

3. **Bring your attention to your feet.** Notice how they feel on the ground, or how your socks feel against your skin. Bring awareness to any sensations you feel in your feet and toes, without judging them as good or bad. As you inhale, follow the breath from your nose to your lungs, down into your belly, and through to your legs and toes. Exhale and relax. Follow one more breath down to your feet, noticing any sensations that may arise.

4. **On your next inhale, bring your attention to your legs.** Notice any sensations in your ankles and calves, then your knees and thighs. Observe any soreness or discomfort, without trying to change or judge the sensations. Send another breath through your legs and notice if the sensations change.

5. **On your next inhale, bring your attention to your lower back**. Notice any tension you might be holding in that area of your body and bring your awareness to it.

6. **Follow your breath into your abdomen**. Notice how it rises and falls with each breath.

7. **Focus your breath on your upper back and shoulders**. Notice how these muscles feel. This is a part of the body where many people carry tension. Fill this area with your breath, and as you exhale, notice the points of contact between this area and the surface on which you're sitting or lying.

8. **On your next inhale, feel your breath fill your chest and heart**. Bring your awareness to this area.

9. **On the next inhale, follow your breath to your hands and arms**. Feel the breath flow through your fingers, palms, wrists, and forearms, up to your arms and into your shoulders. Be aware of the sensations in your arms and any thoughts or urges that go with them. If your mind wanders, gently bring your attention back to this area of your body.

10. **Let your attention shift to your head and face**. As you breathe, notice the sensation of air flowing through your nostrils or the slight itch of a hair on your cheek. Notice if your thoughts or sensations shift as you continue to breathe.

11. **Focus on your whole body**. Follow your breath from the top of your head to the tip of your toes and back up.

12. **As you reach the end of this practice, begin to shift awareness from your bodily sensations to the outside world.** Notice any sounds or smells and the texture of the surface on which you are sitting. When you are ready, gently open your eyes.

TIP:

Eventually, with practice, you won't need the script because you'll get used to checking in with your body and releasing any tension that you find.

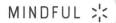

VISUALIZATION: THOUGHTS ON A TRAIN

USEFUL FOR: Bringing awareness to your
thoughts; getting out of rumination

TIME: 2 minutes

It's normal to get caught up in your thoughts, but doing so too often
can take you away from the present moment. If you find yourself
ruminating on or overthinking a problem, this visualization can help
you ground in the here and now by creating some distance between
you and these troublesome thoughts. After all, just because you have
a thought does not make it true.

1. **Find a comfortable place to sit and start paying attention
   to your thoughts.**
2. **Imagine you are sitting on a train and looking out the
   window, watching the scenery go by.** You watch trees and
   houses slip by and people going about their day.
3. **Imagine that these images—these people, places, and
   things you see—are actually the thoughts in your mind.**
   Imagine that your thoughts are just the towns you pass through
   on this train ride.

4. **Notice which thoughts cause an emotional response and which thoughts are just random statements with no emotions attached.** Anger might shout, "My parents are trying to ruin my life!" You have thousands of thoughts a day swirling around you, such as: "What's my mom making for dinner?" "That's a red car." "My nose looks so big today." "It's going to rain." "My friends don't like me." Watch those thoughts go by as you look out the train window.

5. **Notice how even the strongest thoughts or emotions eventually fade, like a town disappearing into the distance.** As you're on a train, you can't get off to visit the towns or talk to the people. Your job is to simply sit back and observe the scenery through the window.

TIP:

This visualization of thoughts passing by can take on many forms. You can imagine thoughts as clouds passing in the sky, or bubbles drifting off, or floats and musicians marching in a parade, or another image that works for you.

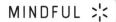

SETTLING YOUR MIND

USEFUL FOR: Nonjudgmental awareness

TIME: 2 minutes

EQUIPMENT: A snow globe. If you don't have one
lying around, you can make your own. Grab a small jar,
fill it with water, and add some glitter. Cover tightly.

Picture a snow globe: The minute you pick it up, the glitter and
sand inside stirs, making it hard to see exactly what is inside. Once
those flakes begin to settle, the water clears and you can see the
figures inside the globe with a lot more clarity. Our minds are a lot
like a snow globe. To clearly see what is going on, you often need to
wait for things to settle.

1. **Pick up the snow globe and shake it a bit.** Observe how the
   flakes stir chaotically in the water.
2. **Watch the glitter as it settles.** Notice how some flakes settle
   quickly, while others take more time to land on the bottom.
   Observe how, with time, the snow globe clears and settles. The
   glitter in the jar represents the thoughts, emotions, and urges
   swirling around in your mind. Through nonjudgmental, watch-

ful attention, these thoughts and urges will settle naturally. Notice that you cannot force the flakes to settle any faster than they do. The same way the flakes do not settle at the same speed, some thoughts take longer to settle than others. It's only with patience that you can allow your mind to fully settle at its own pace.

3. **When the glitter settles, check in with your mind.** Is it more settled than before you tried this exercise? Know that it can take longer for your mind to settle than for glitter to land on the bottom of a snow globe. If you need, flip the jar or globe over and watch the flakes settle again.

TIP:

Know that it's normal if your mind wanders. That makes you human. If you start thinking about how stupid or boring this task is, rephrase it as "I'm having the thought that this is stupid or boring." This is a gentle way to refocus on the task of paying attention to your thoughts.

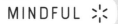

SQUARE BREATHING

USEFUL FOR: Everyday relaxation

TIME: 2 minutes

This is another quick mindfulness strategy to add to your toolbox. The more strategies you have that work for you, the easier it will be to pull one out when you need it. As with other mindfulness skills, it can help refocus your mind and calm down your body when you're feeling anxious. This breathing technique can be used when you are stressed and need a moment of calm, or as an extended meditation when you have more time.

1. **Find a comfortable position.**
2. **Slowly inhale for four seconds.**
3. **Hold your breath for four seconds.**
4. **Slowly exhale for four seconds.**
5. **Hold your breath for four seconds.**
6. **Repeat this cycle four times.**

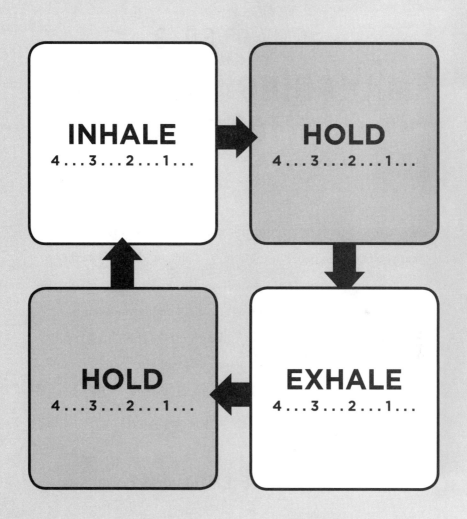

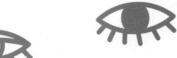
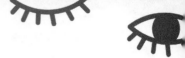

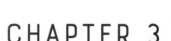

CHAPTER 3

MANAGING DIFFICULT EMOTIONS

Negative emotions can be difficult to tease apart. You might know that you're feeling bad, but might not be able to identify whether you're annoyed, angry, sad, or anxious. This experience is totally normal—it can be hard to distinguish challenging emotions because they often impact and play off each other. This chapter will focus on anger, sadness, and depression. It will offer practical tools for accepting these challenging emotions, and strategies for when you feel stuck in negativity.

WHAT ARE EMOTIONS?

Emotions are big and messy, and we have them all the time. When I ask anyone—both adults and teens—what emotions are, they typically have a tough time answering. Sure, they can name feelings, but that's not the same as understanding them.

Any emotion, positive or negative, can be broken down into that "thought-sensation-behavior" CBT model. No emotion is "bad," because each emotion has a purpose—to give us information so we can make decisions about how to seek safety. Each emotion is connected to an action, and that action is somehow adaptive; that is, it's a reaction to what we're feeling.

Think about your own hardwired fears. If a tiger showed up at your door right this minute, you'd be afraid. That's your emotion. Because of that emotion, you would want to run away as fast as you can or slam the door on the tiger to defend yourself. This action would keep you safe, which is good. All emotions have this type of adaptive action built in. When you're happy, you want to keep doing whatever's making you happy so you can increase your happiness. When you're sad, you want to cry or be alone so you can process. When you're angry, you want to defend yourself.

DEALING WITH ANGER

When was the last time you felt angry? I'm sure it wasn't so long ago. It's normal to feel angry or irritable. Anger is adaptive. If you never felt angry, you'd probably let people walk all over you. Anger prompts us to defend our rights, which can be a good thing. The problem comes when it rules the day and makes you act out in ways you may later regret. Picture this: Two of your best friends post a picture on Instagram showing them having a great time hanging out, and you weren't invited. You feel yourself getting furious. Your face gets hot and you think, "The nerve of them! They're such jerks for going out without me!" You text them and curse them out in ALL CAPS about how selfish they are. You find out later that they did invite you but you missed the text message. You're not sure how to take back what you said.

Anger is normal; it's not good or bad. But the way you act on it can have consequences. You can't take back angry texts, undo aggression, or make a teacher forget that you cursed at them for not giving you an extension. It's important to figure out when it's productive to act on your anger—like standing up for your rights or the rights of others—and when it will just get you into trouble. It's tempting to argue that anger is something you can't control, but that's beside the point. You're right that you can't switch your feelings on or off, but just because you *feel* angry doesn't mean you need to *act* on that feeling. You're in control of your actions.

It can be helpful to figure out what triggers your anger so you can prepare yourself for situations where you might get angry. Try using the mood tracking skills in the "Uncovering Your Triggers" section (PAGE 19). You can also try some of the mindfulness exercises in the previous chapter.

FIND THE ROOT OF YOUR ANGER

What angers you? Finding your triggers can help you stop your anger cycle earlier and learn how to cope. Take a few minutes to think about your triggers. Remember, they don't need to be actions or events. Triggers can also be words, thoughts, or even bodily sensations. To figure out what sets you off, think back to a time when you felt angry. Ask yourself these questions:

- **Was I hurt physically or emotionally?**
- **Were my expectations not met?**
- **Were my needs not met?**
- **Was there something specific about the situation that made me angry—like a person, sound, or sight?**
- **What was I thinking or doing before I started feeling angry?**
- **Was I triggered by something in the past rather than the present situation?**

Anger is an emotional response to not feeling safe, or to needs not being met. This is especially true in close relationships, like with friends or family, where you think they should know better than to do what they did or say what they said. When it feels like an emotional safety barrier is breached, it can feel like the other person betrayed you or broke their part of a contract.

Your thoughts contribute a lot to your anger triggers. Consider again past situations where you felt angry. Did any of these types of thoughts run through your mind?

- "That person caused me harm or made fun of me."
- "That person hurt me on purpose."
- "That person 'should have' acted differently or known better."

It's important to know your triggers, and the thoughts that follow, because this knowledge can help you identify good coping skills. Remember again that *feeling* angry is normal, but acting on this feeling can damage your relationships and leave you feeling emotionally drained.

DEALING WITH SADNESS AND DEPRESSION

Sadness is another challenging emotion. Even though it's normal for everyone to feel sad sometimes, it can be very unpleasant, and extreme sadness can be a symptom of depression. Psychologists are trained to recognize when sadness has turned into depression. Here are some questions to distinguish between depression and normal sadness that comes with being a teenager:

- **Are you sad more days than not?**
- **Have you lost interest in activities that used to make you happy?**
- **Do you feel irritable almost every day?**

If your sadness is persistent and lasts for two weeks, or if you've felt like a black cloud has been hanging over you for a year, you might be depressed, not just sad. To meet the criteria for a diagnosis of depression, psychologists look for specific changes in things like appetite (increased or decreased eating), sleep (trouble falling asleep or sleeping too much), focus (trouble concentrating or feeling that your mind goes blank), and energy level (trouble getting yourself going or feeling fidgety). Psychologists also look for changes in thoughts. Do you feel hopeless about yourself, your abilities, and your future? Do you often feel guilty? We also know that with teens, depression can show up as irritability or grouchiness. If you're experiencing many of these symptoms, you might be dealing with depression.

Remember how every emotion is connected to an action? Sadness makes you want to withdraw. It makes you want to stay alone in your room, play video games, pull the covers over your head, and totally disconnect. This can feel good in the moment—if you're depressed and take a nap, at least you don't feel anything while you're asleep. Eventually, though, you wake up. And you often feel even worse once you do. You might turn down your friends' invitation to go out, then feel awful when they all post pictures of themselves hanging out without you. And since now you missed the inside jokes, you feel even more removed from them. Depression brings on

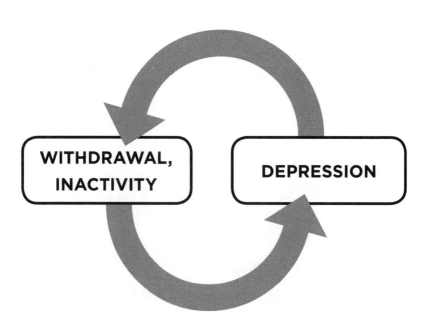

a cycle of inactivity: You do nothing, so you feel bad, and because you feel bad, you do even less, which makes you feel even worse.

Instead of giving in to the impulse to withdraw, the best way to manage depressed feelings is to take away its power by *not* acting on it. The skills in this chapter can help keep sadness from taking full control, and with practice you can take steps to reverse the depressive cycle.

If you are depressed, you might wish you were dead or have thoughts about what the world would be like without you. You might think of hurting or killing yourself. Suicidal thoughts are a serious symptom of depression. If you are feeling this way, know that there are people trained to support you through emotional crisis. You can text "HOME" to 741741 or call 1-800-273-TALK (8255) 24 hours a day, seven days a week, to speak with someone who can help.

SITTING WITH YOUR EMOTIONS

Do you know why it's so hard not to react when you feel an intense emotion, even if you know, logically, that acting on it may not be the best choice? It's because emotions tell us that if we don't respond to them *right now*, they'll never go away on their own. But this is totally false. Though sometimes they feel like tornados, emotions are more like waves that ebb and flow. They come on strong, but eventually, if you give them time, they go away on their own.

The best way to allow challenging emotions to come and go is to accept them. Acceptance doesn't mean you agree with or give in to the emotions; it just means you acknowledge that they exist. Denying or refusing to acknowledge them can come back to hit you in the face. Attending to difficult emotions, on the other hand, will help you get over them faster without the long-term side effects of avoidance.

When you're in the thick of an intense negative emotion, it can be hard to know what to do. The skills on the following pages are meant to give you tools to teach you to work through and sit with your emotions, so you can better cope with your depression, anger, and anxiety.

SET SMALL GOALS

USEFUL FOR: Getting yourself motivated
to change your depressed mood

TIME: Varies, but daily

Depression zaps energy and makes it harder to do things that used to be easy. Setting small goals can help break the cycle of inactivity and withdrawal, getting you back to a healthier routine. The idea is to build a foundation of healthy habits that can help improve your mood, like self-care and exercise. Don't set large, ambitious goals that set you up for disappointment. You'll feel better if you pick small goals that are manageable and realistic but still move you in a positive direction. Once you feel the positive effects of these little steps, you might feel motivated to take bigger ones.

SELF-CARE:

Have you gotten out of the habit of brushing your teeth, showering, or cleaning your room? Reintroducing these self-care activities can improve your mood by helping you feel a little bit better about yourself. If a task feels too overwhelming, break it down into small, doable steps and set a time frame so it won't feel endless. Let's take the example of a messy bedroom. Instead of trying to clean it all up in one day, try this approach:

1. **Set the goal of cleaning up just one part of the room each day, for 15 minutes a day.**
2. **Break down what needs to get done into simpler 15-minute tasks, for example: picking up clothes, vacuuming, sorting papers, etc.**
3. **Tackle each of these tasks individually.** Take one day to pick up the clothes, another day to go through papers, another day to vacuum. In this way, you see a little improvement each day but don't feel too bogged down with the chore.
4. **Remember that no step is too small.** Just hanging up your coat when you've gotten into the habit of dumping it on the ground can be a huge step forward!

EXERCISE:

We know movement is an effective way to get out of a bad mood, but it can be hard to work out when you're feeling depressed. Like cleaning your room, you don't want to set goals that are too hard or overwhelming. Don't start off by saying you're going to jog for an hour five days a week. Instead, try the steps on the following page.

1. **Set the target of walking around the block for five minutes before school, just one day a week.** This might seem too insignificant to make a difference, but it's a small step you can consistently build on.

2. **The following week, try doing 10 minutes, and the week after that, 15.** Or if you want to keep it at 5 minutes, just add a second walk to the week. Eventually you might feel energized enough by these short walks to turn them into short jogs. Small changes can have big effects here. Even putting on your sneakers and workout clothes can be a step in the right direction.

3. **Pick a type of exercise you enjoy.** If you like basketball, try shooting hoops for 10 minutes. If dance is your thing, play one song you love and dance in your room. To get motivated, just get moving!

TIP:
If you don't see any change in your mood right away, that's OK. Celebrate the success of doing something you wouldn't have done before, and do it again tomorrow.

PLAN ACTIVITIES YOU VALUE

USEFUL FOR: Reversal of depression's cycle of withdrawal

TIME: You decide, but take time each day or week to plan in advance. A good initial target for an activity is 30 minutes a day.

When you're feeling depressed, it's easy to withdraw from people and activities that were once important to you. The exercise below will help you identify activities that bring value and joy to your life, so you can feel more energized and accomplished.

1. **Make a list of activities you once enjoyed or that you might enjoy trying.** The best ones are the ones that get you moving. They can range from simple activities, like going to the movies, to ones that require more planning, like an art project or going for a hike (getting some sun is always a good option!). Have some options that are simple for you to achieve, and others that are more ambitious. Think of things that can be done solo or at home, like making a playlist of music to listen to, and others that involve friends or family, like playing board games or

sports. Approach this like a brainstorm—there are no wrong answers, and the longer the list, the better, because you'll have more options to choose from.

2. **Once you have a list of options, pick one that feels doable and make a plan.** The more specific, the better. Think about how you can incorporate it into your day, when you're going to do it, and how long you're going to spend doing it. For example, if baking is on your list, think about when and what you'll be baking—"On Monday night around 8 p.m. I'm going to make chocolate chip cookies," or "I'm going to go for a half-hour walk after school on Monday and Wednesday."

3. **Give yourself weekly targets.** Think about what might get in the way of those goals. You can even consider giving yourself a little reward if you meet those goals!

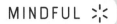
SELF-SOOTHING

USEFUL FOR: Being able to "ride the
wave" of uncomfortable emotions

TIME: Varies

Self-soothing is a good skill when you feel completely overwhelmed by your feelings. Emotions fade with time, so it's a way to buy time. When your emotions start feeling more manageable, you can move on to other mindful skills. In this exercise, you'll choose five activities for each of your five senses to calm and comfort yourself. I've provided some examples for each.

1. **Vision:** Go for a walk and look around at the trees or flowers; watch a movie trailer or silly video.

2. **Hearing:** Listen to a calming song that you like; listen to nature and notice what you can hear around you.

3. **Touch:** Take a bath and notice how your body feels in the water.

4. **Taste:** Treat yourself to a special snack. Eat it slowly and savor each bite.

5. **Smell:** Notice the smells around you. Sniff your favorite perfume or a food you love.

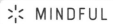

LISTEN TO YOUR EMOTIONS

USEFUL FOR: Feeling in control of your emotions
(rather than having them control you!)

TIME: 2 to 5 minutes

Even the most intense emotions vary in intensity from moment to moment. One way to cope with challenging emotions is to notice them, be able to label them, and sit with them. When you're able to intentionally focus your attention on what's around you, you may feel more in control.

1. **Using the general mindfulness rules of observation and description, notice what emotions you're experiencing.** Rate them on a scale of 0 to 10, with 10 being the most intense.
2. **Observe what your body feels like while it's experiencing the emotion.** Are your muscles heavy? Does your face feel warm?
3. **Describe these physical feelings to yourself using three statements or more.**
4. **Turn your attention to your thoughts.** Notice what they are without judging them. Observe them like a scientist in a lab, without trying to change or influence them.

5. **Keep watching to see if there are any changes in the intensity of your thoughts, emotions, or physical sensations as you observe them.** If your attention wanders, just bring it back to the exercise without judging yourself for losing focus.

TIP:

If this skill feels uncomfortable at first, that's normal. When was the last time you sat and let yourself experience uncomfortable emotions for two minutes?

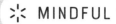

ABDOMINAL BREATHING

USEFUL FOR: Reducing stress and anger

TIME: 1 minute a day until you're used to
it, then when you feel stressed

In moments of high stress, it can be helpful to take a step back and relax your body. You might have noticed that your breathing gets shallow when you're feeling anxious, as if air doesn't completely fill your lungs. Under stress we often don't breathe with our diaphragm (the muscle under our ribs that pulls air in and out), which can make us light-headed or dizzy and cause even more distress. Even though breathing is automatic, it can be controlled.

1. **Lie on your back or sit comfortably in a chair.** Close your eyes if that's comfortable for you, or focus on a spot in front of you.

2. **Put one hand on your chest and the other on your belly.** Notice which hand moves as you breathe normally (it's usually the one on your chest).

3. **Breathe in slowly through your nose.** As you inhale, picture your belly filling with air like a balloon. Feel it press against your hand.

4. **Breathe out slowly through your mouth.** As you exhale, picture that balloon deflating and feel your belly sink in, almost like you're pulling your belly button toward your spine.

5. **Repeat.** As you breathe in, feel your belly fill with air. The hand on your chest should stay relatively still. As you exhale, feel your belly relax and fall inward. Try not to tense your stomach muscles; just let the breath fill your body naturally through your nose and into your lungs. Let it leave your body the same way, without forcing it. This exercise works best when you exhale for longer than you inhale.

TIP:

Some teens with anxiety find this type of relaxation uncomfortable. That's OK and normal. It can still be useful to be aware of our breath and to learn how to take calming breaths, even if they're initially not so calming. A good time to practice this skill is in bed before going to sleep.

WRITE IT OUT

USEFUL FOR: Anger reduction

TIME: 15 minutes

A little self-awareness can go a long way when you're angry. Anger often encourages quick action or reaction. This skill gets you to slow down and consider the consequences before acting.

When you notice yourself feeling angry, write down responses to these prompts.

- **Why am I angry? What are my thoughts? What do I feel in my body? What do I want to do with this emotion?**
- **What are the consequences of acting the way I want to act? What would happen if I acted this way?**
- **Are there any alternatives I can try instead? (Write down one or two.)**
- **What are the consequences of those alternative actions? (Think them through.)**

Make a choice based on your analysis. Often, the best choice is one that is "good enough," but not perfect. That's OK; notice what happens when you make this choice.

Here's an example of this skill:
Juan is fuming because his dad told him he couldn't go out until he finished all his homework. He identifies anger as his core emotion and recognizes that he's thinking, "This is just so unfair!!!" His face gets hot. His muscles tense up. He really wants to play video games to spite his dad. He thinks about the consequences: If he blows off all his homework, he'll probably get in more trouble. That would mean even less time with friends. He lays out a couple alternatives: He can suck it up and do his work, or he can try to negotiate a deal. If he did all his work, he'd get to go out, but it might be late to catch a movie with friends and he'd probably be mad about "letting his dad win." Then he thinks about negotiating. His dad is normally reasonable, so maybe he can ask to go out after finishing his math homework if he promises to do the rest when he comes home. He decides to act on this last choice.

TIP:
Compare when you get angry and use this skill to times when you get angry and don't. Notice any difference? Doing the opposite of your instinct is often a good alternative. If your anger wants you to lash out and yell, you can speak in a calm voice, go for a walk, or even apologize. This can help lessen the tension of a situation instead of making it worse.

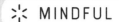

BE KIND TO YOURSELF

USEFUL FOR: When challenging emotions
make you feel down on yourself

TIME: 1 minute a day

Challenging emotions can take a toll on your self-esteem by making you feel bad about how you're feeling, bringing on even more negative emotions like shame or guilt. This is especially true of depression, but it applies to anger and anxiety as well.

1. **Think about what you tell yourself when you're struggling with a task because of your anxiety, depression, or anger.** Do you ever tell yourself that you totally suck at the task at hand? Or that you're a total failure and must be the only one having trouble? If you do, you're not alone. We're often our own worst critic.

2. **Consider what you would tell a friend who was struggling with a similar situation.** Would you be as harsh on them? What would you tell them? Would you comfort them? Encourage them?

3. **Take a moment to offer these kind words to yourself.**

4. **Think about something nice you can do for yourself.**

5. **Give yourself a break.** Can you reframe your perceived failures as something a bit more kind? If, for example, you're having a hard time with this exercise, instead of insulting yourself, say something like "It's hard to do something right the first time. I'm learning. Maybe I'll get it next time." Like all the other skills, being gentle with yourself will take dedication and practice.

TIP:

Try making this a part of your morning routine. Tell yourself kind, supportive words while you're getting dressed or brushing your teeth. It can feel awkward to be kind to yourself when you're not used to it, so you may need to try multiple times before you get feel comfortable.

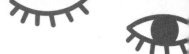

CHAPTER 4

CHANGING YOUR THOUGHTS

Anxiety changes the way you see the world. The sky may be blue, but if you're wearing tinted sunglasses, it'll look different from reality. Your thoughts do the same thing: They take reality, filter it, and sometimes distort it through emotions like anxiety or anger.

This chapter will help you recognize some common thought patterns that make anxiety worse. Once you're able to recognize them, you can apply strategies to help you think in a healthier, more balanced way.

ACCEPTING YOUR THOUGHTS

Your brain is filled with noise. Take a minute to pay attention to the thoughts running through your head. You can try using the "Realistic Thoughts" skill (PAGE 106) as a starting point. What did you notice?

Thoughts can be positive ("Hey, this is a great exercise!"), neutral ("This book is blue"), or negative ("I'll never master this skill!"). The thoughts that pop up instinctively or without you even noticing are called your automatic thoughts. When automatic thoughts are negative, they can suck you into a toxic loop.

If you make a mistake and think to yourself, "There I go again, messing everything up!" you're going to feel even worse, which will only increase your negative thinking and create an overwhelming, self-inflicted cycle. It's easy to get trapped in your thoughts. My aim isn't necessarily to change your thoughts—it's to help you change your *relationship* to those thoughts so they don't take over and make you more anxious.

STICKY MIND

Imagine this scenario: You see a friend walking down the street. He passes you without saying hi. What thoughts go through your mind? Here are some possibilities:

"He's such a jerk! Why is he ignoring me?!"

"I guess I'm not cool enough for him to acknowledge me."

"Oh well, I guess he didn't see me."

What you think will play a large role in how you feel. If your automatic thought is "He's such a jerk!" you'll probably feel angry. If it's "I guess I'm not cool," you'll probably feel sad or self-conscious. And if your automatic thought is "I guess he didn't see me," you'll probably just keep on walking without feeling much.

People tend to remember negative thoughts more than neutral or positive ones. Thoughts like "My shoes are red" or "School starts at 7:20 a.m." come and go, but thoughts like "None of my friends like me" have a lot more power. They stick. Once a thought makes you anxious, you notice it more and try to unstick it. And when you try to unstick it, it gets even more stuck.

Here's a mini-experiment: For the next minute, think about anything at all *but* a dancing pink elephant. Anything. Chances are that before you read that sentence, you weren't thinking about elephants at all. But now you probably have a bunch of pink elephants dancing in your head.

All you need to do is mention something weird for it to stick, and trying to unstick only makes it stick more. Remember that negative emotions are like quicksand—the more you move around, the deeper and quicker you sink. The more you try and fight these thoughts, the more they stick, and the more power they get. So how do you change sticky thoughts? The first step is to notice the common tricks our minds play on us.

THINKING TRAPS

Your brain is designed to take shortcuts. This is normal and healthy—it's what makes humans great thinkers and inventors! But it also means that your mind will sometimes connect two things that are not related or see things in a way that isn't very helpful. These unhelpful thinking patterns can put you in more distress, so being able to identify them is an important step toward more positive thinking. Here's a list of the most common types of thinking errors, or "thinking traps," that contribute to negative emotions. As you read through them, notice which ones you relate to most.

ALL OR NOTHING

This type of black-and-white thinking means you tend to see everything in extremes, ignoring anything in the middle. If you aren't perfect, you might see yourself as a complete failure. For example, you might think, "I can't believe I got a 90 on that exam! I'm such a failure—I'll never get into college!" or "Ugh, I'm feeling sad again today—I'll never ever be happy." The truth is normally somewhere in between. A 90 is still a good grade and probably will not impact your college acceptance. And it's normal to feel sad sometimes, but emotions fade and you will feel happy again.

JUMPING TO CONCLUSIONS

This thinking trap involves forming a negative interpretation of a situation without evidence to support your conclusion. This form of thinking shows up in two main ways:

- **Mind reading:** When you make assumptions about other people's thoughts or motivations, especially related to how they treat you, for example, "My brother meant to hurt me when he closed the door."

- **Fortune-telling:** Predicting that things will go badly in the future, for example, "I'm totally going to bomb this audition."

Instead, reality is more nuanced. It might be true that your brother meant to hurt you, but an alternative view can be that he didn't see you and it was an accident. And yes, there's a chance you will bomb the audition, but if you've gotten important roles in plays before, it's more likely that you will perform well.

CATASTROPHIZING

This involves taking an unpleasant detail or event and blowing things out of proportion by seeing it as a pattern, for example, thinking, "My friends never include me!" when you are excluded once, or "I always lose everything!" when you misplace an item one time. Bad things do happen, but going to the extreme makes you feel worse. An alternative perspective is that though you were excluded, you are mostly included by your friends, or that you sometimes lose things but that's normal.

EMOTIONAL REASONING

This is when you take your own emotional reaction as evidence by believing that because you *feel* a certain way, then what you're thinking must be true. By this logic, if you're feeling anxious at the dentist, then the dentist must be dangerous. Or if you're feeling angry, it must mean that your friend definitely treated you unfairly.

I get anxious at the doctor all the time (I hate shots!), but that isn't proof that my doctor is scary! In fact, she's a really nice woman who is doing her best to keep me healthy, so I do my best to separate the emotion from the facts.

IGNORING THE GOOD

Anytime you do something well, you find a way to twist it so it doesn't count. This is also called "discounting the positive." You might tell yourself that while you aced that one test, it was easy, so anyone could have done well. This negative self-talk will only make you feel like you're never good enough. And it's also false—your good work counts!

This is similar to another error called "magnification." When you look through binoculars, you see only one detail of a larger picture. Here, you "zoom in" on the negative parts rather than seeing the whole situation. You might think, "This whole art project is a failure!" when you get critical feedback on one part of it, even if you get positive feedback on the rest. It's normal to dislike criticism, but wouldn't you feel better if you found a way to zoom out on the positive feedback as well?

"SHOULD" STATEMENTS

Words like "should," "must," or "need to" tend to make you feel bad about yourself or angry at others. These statements often become rigid rules that cause more distress than you might realize. If you think to yourself, "I should have practiced more for that presentation," you're beating yourself up for past mistakes instead of living in the present. If you think, "My friend shouldn't have said that to me," you'll feel unnecessarily angry and resentful about a situation you probably couldn't control. The alternative to "shoulds" is to recognize that things don't always go your way but you can manage more than you think you can. So yes, it would have been nice if your friend was more sensitive to you, but you're still friends and you can move past it.

HOW TO GET UNSTUCK

Do you recognize any of these negative thinking patterns in yourself? Which ones cause you problems or distress? Now that you're beginning to understand more about the relationship between sticky thoughts and difficult emotions, you're ready for the next step. The skills in the next few pages will help you begin shifting your relationship to negative thoughts and emotions by:

- **Recognizing that you are not your thoughts**
- **Challenging your automatic thoughts, recognizing your thinking errors, and developing healthier ways of thinking about difficult situations**

Changing your thoughts can be hard. You've probably been falling into thinking traps for a while, and at first it might be tough to catch them. With practice, however, you can create new thinking patterns. Here's an example:

Marina always felt anxious about hanging out with kids from school. She worried that no one liked her and that the girls in her class were "too cool" for her. When they did hang out, she never disagreed with them for fear that they wouldn't want to spend time with her again. She avoided making plans to avoid getting rejected.

During a therapy session, we focused on recognizing her thinking traps: She often engaged in all-or-nothing thinking, and magnified negative interactions while ignoring positive ones. We worked together to figure out whether it was true that her friends didn't like her. She acknowledged that people did talk to her in school and even texted her to make plans. Even when she fought with them, they seemed to go back to treating her like a friend the next day. So we developed coping statements that she could tell herself whenever she noticed anxious thoughts arise. Instead of falling for the automatic thoughts about being disliked, she began to think, "I do have friends—even if I fight with them sometimes." Whenever she noticed a particularly sticky thought, she used mindfulness and acceptance to recognize that her thoughts are just thoughts and not the absolute truth.

HEALTHY THINKING SKILLS

Healthy thinking is not the same as positive thinking. Negative experiences happen—getting sick, losing house keys, fighting with friends—and negative thoughts and emotions are a normal part of those experiences. Healthy thinking doesn't mean taking an unrealistically positive approach to everything; it means taking in the whole picture, both the good and the bad. For example, thinking, "Driving is hard, and I'm going to need to practice until I get it," is very different from thinking, "Driving is impossible, and I'll never learn to parallel park; my parents will be driving me around forever." The first thought isn't positive, but it is a realistic view of the situation.

The first step to healthy thinking begins with awareness of your automatic thoughts, which you'll learn in the exercise, "Analyzing Your Thoughts" on the following page. You'll learn to identify your thoughts, label your thinking traps, and weigh the evidence to figure out if your thoughts are correct. From there, you'll be introduced to other skills that will help you handle sticky thoughts and negative self-talk as well as cope with challenging situations.

ANALYZING YOUR THOUGHTS

USEFUL FOR: Untwisting thoughts that make you anxious

TIME: Formally once a day, but can be done
informally anytime you feel anxious

EQUIPMENT: A notebook or journal

If you can name your thoughts, you can identify thinking traps and use skills to reduce your anxious thinking. Your goal is to separate these anxious thoughts from your emotions and behaviors. This builds on the "Monitor Your Thoughts, Feelings, and Behaviors" (PAGE 25) by taking a deeper dive into your thoughts.

~~~~~~~~~~~~~~~~~~~~~~~~

STEP 1: IDENTIFY YOUR THOUGHTS

Turn to a new page in your notebook. Divide it into three columns, leaving some extra space at the top of the page above the columns (see PAGE 101). There are three parts to this skill—this first one will only use the first column.

Now, think about a difficult emotion you're currently experiencing or have recently experienced. In the space above the columns, write down the emotion.

Just below that, describe the situation. Write a few lines about what happened using the following questions as guides:

a. **What are the facts? Who was there, and what happened?**

b. **If I took a photo of the situation, what would I see? Pictures don't lie, so this can be a good way to separate what you felt from what happened.**

c. **What emotions did I feel in this situation?**

Move down to the first column and label it "My thoughts." This is where you write down the thoughts running in your head during the situation. Ask yourself, "If I was in a comic book and there was a thought bubble above my head, what would it say?" Jot that down.

STEP 2: LABEL IT

The next step to healthy thinking is identifying any thinking traps. Ask yourself, "Am I falling into a thinking trap here? Do my thoughts fit into any of these categories?" Chances are, if you're feeling bad, there's some kind of thinking trap present.

Label the second column "Thinking trap" and write down any traps you might recognize. Don't stress too much about making sure you list the "right" thinking trap. Many thoughts can fit into more than one trap. The important thing is to approach your thoughts with an observant eye.

STEP 3: EXAMINE THE EVIDENCE

This step will help you evaluate your thoughts and determine if they are actually true. Take your thought and treat it like a scientist would. Label the third column "Evidence" and fill it in with the answers to the questions below. Then identify an alternative thought based on your evidence.

a. **What proof do I have that this thought is true?**

b. **Is there any evidence that this thought might not be true? What is it? Try to list as much evidence as you can.**

c. **What's the probability that the thing I fear will come true?**

TIP:

Be aware that sometimes a situation really is negative. When you face those situations, you can focus on acceptance and coping. You're more resilient than you realize, and can deal with a lot more than you might expect.

EXAMPLE:

EMOTION: Worried

SITUATION: I walked into my house, and it was really quiet.
I didn't hear my mom or my dog.

MY THOUGHTS	THINKING TRAP	EVIDENCE	
Something bad happened to my mom. Maybe she was kidnapped while I was at school.	Jumping to conclusions; catastrophizing	**Evidence for "Something bad happened to my mom."** • She's normally around when I get home. • She normally texts me when she's late.	**Evidence against "Something bad happened to my mom."** • I don't know anyone who has ever been kidnapped. • Sometimes she's late and doesn't have time to let me know. • She might be in the backyard or taking the dog for a walk, and that's why I don't hear her.

COPING STATEMENTS

USEFUL FOR: Developing healthy thinking

TIME: Formally once a day, but can be done informally anytime you feel anxious

EQUIPMENT: Notebook or journal

You have now identified your thoughts, labeled your thinking traps, and weighed the evidence to figure out if your thoughts are correct. It's time to pull it all together and come up with ways to handle challenging situations. One powerful tool to keep in your toolbox is "coping statements"—phrases you can tell yourself when automatic thoughts pop up. When you focus on coping, your worry loses some of its power. Use this skill to finish up the "thinking skills" chart you started earlier.

1. **Using the proof you came up with in "Step 3: Examine the Evidence" in the previous exercise, ask yourself some questions:**

   - Is there any other way for me to think about this situation based on the evidence I have?
   - Is my initial thought the only possibility here?

- If I thought about this situation in a different way, would I be less anxious?
- If this same situation happened to my friend, what would I tell them?
- If the situation I fear actually happened, could I cope with it?

2. **Based on your answers, come up with a simple statement that responds to the automatic thoughts by framing the situation in a more realistic and helpful way.** This is your coping statement. In the example above, your coping statement might be: "It's really, really unlikely that she would be kidnapped. She's probably just somewhere I can't hear her."

TIP:

Coping statements don't always "feel" true when you first start to use them. Think about how many times you've thought your automatic thoughts—dozens, hundreds, maybe a thousand times! All automatic thoughts, even unhealthy ones, are like well-worn sneakers. They just "fit." New thoughts are like a new pair of shoes. You need to break them in before they feel comfortable. So stick with the coping thought for at least a week or two before making any decisions about whether or not it works for you.

WORRY TIME

USEFUL FOR: Limiting your worried thoughts

TIME: 10 minutes a day

EQUIPMENT: Notebook or journal

Anxious thoughts try to take over all your thinking. Sometimes it can feel like the minute you knock down one worried thought, there's another one waiting right behind it. This strategy focuses on postponing your worries by setting up a time when you can worry all you want. You might find that this decreases your overall anxiety and helps you regain control over your life.

1. **Pick a 10-minute period that will be your "worry time."**
2. **When a worry comes up over the course of the day outside of this worry time, very briefly jot down the issue or situation and any triggers.** Since it's not your official worry time, refocus your full attention on what you're doing.
3. **When your worry time comes, pull out your list and dig in!** Think about your worries as much as you can. This isn't a time for solutions. If you get bored, notice that feeling—and note if it surprises you.

4. If you catch yourself still going over the same worries after your worry time, just write it down and think about it during your worry time tomorrow.

TIP:

It's not a great idea to schedule worry time for right before you go to bed, since the anxiety can keep you from falling asleep. Find a time during the day. If you think you need more time to focus on your worries, you can try setting two daily worry periods, for example, one in the morning and one in the afternoon, or you can make a longer, 20-minute period.

ACTION 4

REALISTIC THOUGHTS

USEFUL FOR: Reality-checking your worried thoughts

TIME: As needed

EQUIPMENT: Notebook or journal

It can be hard to judge your anxious thoughts for what they are. We all have a negative voice inside our head that sometimes pulls us down or tells us situations are more dangerous than they really are. This skill focuses on identifying realistic alternatives to your anxious thoughts. Realistic thinking is healthy thinking because it looks at the whole picture instead of looking only at your anxiety's warped view of a situation.

1. **After you've identified your thoughts and labeled any thinking traps, evaluate your evidence and come to some conclusions:**

   - Have I confused a fact with an opinion?
   - Am I 100 percent sure my thought is true?
   - Am I confusing something possible for something that will definitely happen?

2. If you're not sure about these answers, here are a few additional strategies for reality-checking yourself:

- Poll your friends (in real life or social media) about what they would do or think.
- Look online. This is not something I often suggest, but if you want to determine how realistic your worries are, you can Google the likelihood of being bitten by a shark or struck by lightning. (Spoiler: You're way more likely to get hurt by almost anything else than get bitten by a shark!)
- Create a summary statement that you can tell yourself when this worry comes up. Write out a more realistic thought based on the evidence and facts you've uncovered. This should be a go-to "reality check" of your fear. For example, include statistics about shark bites!

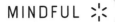

SING YOUR THOUGHTS

USEFUL FOR: Taking the power away from anxious thoughts

TIME: 2 minutes

You might have a particularly strong, sticky thought that you just can't shake or reality-check away. That inner critic may be constantly berating you with thoughts like "You're so stupid" or "No one wants to be your friend." This skill can help you treat your thoughts as what they are—oftentimes silly, meaningless words!

1. **Identify your sticky thought.**
2. **Sing it to a familiar tune like "Old MacDonald Had a Farm" or "Happy Birthday."** Instead of singing, you can also try saying your thoughts in a cartoonish voice.
3. **Notice if repeating the thought over and over this way helps it lose its grip on you.**

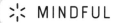
BE YOUR OWN FRIEND

USEFUL FOR: Finding compassion for yourself

TIME: 5 minutes a day

EQUIPMENT: Notebook or journal

All that negative self-talk can have an impact on your self-esteem and overall well-being. You probably wouldn't speak to a friend the way you so often speak to yourself. This exercise is designed to help you practice self-compassion by putting someone else in your shoes. In your notebook, write down the answers to the prompts below.

1. **Think about a time when a good friend was struggling.**

   - How would you support this friend?
   - What would you do for them?
   - What would you say, and what tone would you use?

2. **Now think of yourself and your own struggles.** It could be with anxiety or anything else. How did you treat yourself? What thoughts or judgments ran through your head? What did you say to yourself, and what tone did you use?

3. **Notice any differences between these two responses.** How do you respond to your friend's struggles differently than you respond to your own?

4. **Think about how your thoughts, feelings, and behaviors might change if you responded to your own struggles in the way you would respond to a friend's—even by just changing the tone of your self-talk.** The next time you notice that you're being unkind to yourself while you're struggling, try talking and acting the way you would with someone you care deeply about.

TIP:

Don't be surprised if this exercise feels weird. When was the last time you practiced some self-compassion? Try it every day for a week and see what happens.

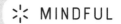

THOUGHTS ON A RIVER

USEFUL FOR: Separating yourself
from your anxious thoughts

TIME: 5 minutes

You are not your thoughts. Sometimes when a thought is particularly sticky, you may find that it's harder to reality-check a situation. Mindfulness practices can help you stay in the present moment so you can separate yourself from your thoughts instead of getting caught up in them.

1. **Close your eyes and take a few deep breaths. Focus your attention on your breathing.**
2. **Imagine a river rushing and swirling in front of you.**
3. **Notice how the river carries everything in its path downstream.** There are pebbles, leaves, muck, and branches, all being carried away. Watch how some leaves drift quickly while others get snagged on rocks. Eventually, though, the river carries them all away.

4. **Imagine the river is your mind, and those leaves, branches, and debris are your thoughts.** As you observe your river, watch your thoughts be carried away. Notice that like leaves, some thoughts do get snagged—that's normal. But also like those leaves on the river, your thoughts eventually drift away. Some thoughts are more uncomfortable than others. Just observe them, without judgment, and you'll see that even these most difficult thoughts do go away with time.

TIP:

Whenever you notice yourself getting overrun by anxious thoughts, you can return to this river, or to any other mindfulness exercise in this book that helps separate you from your thoughts. Remember, practice is key. The more you try, the better you'll be at untangling yourself from these sticky thoughts.

BULLY IN A PLAYGROUND

USEFUL FOR: Separating yourself

from your anxious thoughts

TIME: 5 minutes

When you're stuck in strong, negative beliefs, that critical voice that makes you feel bad about yourself comes out swinging. By recognizing your anxiety bully, you can change your relationship with your thoughts and begin to act differently.

1. **Close your eyes and imagine that your anxiety is a bully.**

   - Bullies get power by getting victims to respond. If a bully says, "You're so ugly!" and you say, "No, I'm not!" then the bully has won. He has the power because he knows he got a good punch at your self-esteem.

   - Instead, respond by not reacting the way they'd expect. If a bully says, "You're so ugly!" and you say, "You're right—I didn't brush my hair this morning," then the bully deflates. Since his power comes from your response, your job is to ignore his insults until he moves on.

2. **Instead of following your anxious thoughts and urges, try nonengagement by allowing them to be present.** If your anxiety tells you, "Hey, you might have a panic attack in math class," try, "I guess that's a possibility."

3. **Know that your anxiety bully might get worse before it gets better.** It makes one last-ditch effort to get your attention when it's being ignored. Sometimes it puts up a fight right at the end, but if you push through it, you'll notice it will start to recede.

TIP:

Give your bully a name to help you recognize when it shows up in your mind. By doing this, you'll be more aware of when your anxiety is trying to get you to think or respond in an unhelpful way, and you'll know it's time to practice non-reacting.

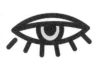

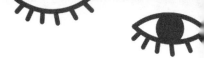

CHAPTER 5

CHALLENGING YOUR BEHAVIORS

Just because you have a thought doesn't mean you have to act on it. Try this: Think to yourself, "I can't read this book." Did it make your brain magically shut down and unable to read? You're probably still reading just fine. Your actions are separate from your thoughts and emotions, so you can choose to act in a way that doesn't automatically respond to them. This chapter will focus on identifying behaviors that can help relieve your anxiety and doing away with the behaviors that get in your way.

ESCAPE AND AVOIDANCE

Anxiety prompts you to escape or avoid a situation. It's as simple as that. If your house is on fire, you're going to want to run away as fast as you can. If you're asked to give an oral presentation, you're also going to want to run away. It's the same automatic response, but the running from fire helps you survive, while running from the classroom doesn't really help. Reducing your avoidance is an important goal in CBT, because avoidance actually makes anxiety worse. Here's an example:

> Marta is afraid of spiders. She thinks they might be poisonous and is creeped out by all their legs. Every time she sees a spider, her body tenses and her breathing speeds up. She runs shrieking out of the room, refusing to go back in until other people assure her that the spider is dead. Her fear is so strong that she decides she no longer wants to go to summer camp. She loves camp and knows she'll miss out on a lot of fun with her friends, but the risk of being around spiders just isn't worth it.

Marta's behavior of running out of the room (her escape response) seems like a good idea at first—she avoids the spider, which is what she wants. That's probably why the next time she sees a spider, she does the same thing and runs away again. It works again, but this behavior pattern ultimately has a negative effect because it just confirms her belief that spiders are dangerous and scary and that she can't handle being in the room with them. The more she runs away, the more she thinks she *needs* to run away to deal with the anxiety. She relies so much on her escape response that she's unable to deal with it on her own, and ends up changing her entire summer plans.

WHY SEEKING SAFETY
ISN'T ALWAYS GOOD

You're afraid. You call your parents. You feel better. Perfect system, right? Not exactly. Calling Mom and Dad to feel safe may sound like a good idea, but anxiety has rebound effects. If you call them to feel calm, you'll *always* have to call them to feel calm. What if they don't pick up, or you're in the middle of something important?

Anxiety is not actually dangerous. But by acting on it, you're basically confirming that it is dangerous. Safety behaviors are anything that calms your anxiety when they don't do anything in reality. Say you think you're having a heart attack, and drink water to get rid of the uncomfortable sensations. Drinking is a safety signal because water doesn't cure heart attacks! Here are other behaviors that may help you feel better in the moment while doing nothing in reality:

- **CHECKING:** This includes making sure locks are locked or stoves are turned off, confirming the location of exits "just in case", or rereading an e-mail more than necessary to make sure it's just right.

- **MENTAL REASSURANCE, MENTAL REVIEW, MENTAL DISTRACTION:** These are tricks you play in your head to make yourself feel better, but reinforce that you can't handle your anxiety without these techniques.

- **SAFETY "STUFF":** Carrying around specific items "just in case." This can be medication that you don't actually need, food, phone numbers, or even needing another person to accompany you.

Avoidance techniques do really help you avoid your anxiety—that's why you keep using them. But our end goal is to cope, not avoid. And these techniques only feed anxiety in the long term!

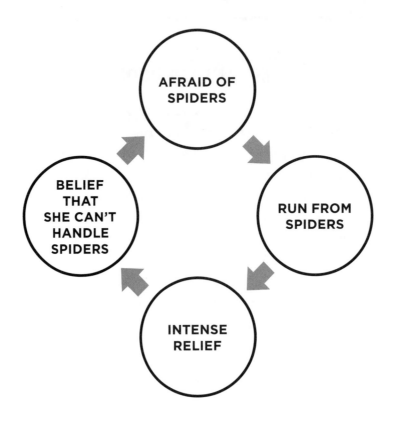

Marta is in a place familiar to many people with anxiety: A certain behavior makes you feel good in the moment but makes your anxiety worse in the long term, because you never learn to coexist with your fear.

WHAT DOES AVOIDANCE LOOK LIKE?

Running away is one obvious manifestation of avoidance, but avoidance can take many forms. You may try to avoid an actual external object in the world or a physical sensation in your body. You might even try to avoid your own thoughts by using distraction or other mental processes.

Here's an example of subtle ways avoidance might show up:

> Malcolm is afraid of death and dying. When the
> topic comes up, he tries to change the subject.
> When he's stuck in a conversation related to sick-
> ness, he thinks about other things. If he hears
> about a sick friend, he goes through a mental
> checklist of ways to know that he's healthy, and
> calls his parents at work to get reassurance that he's
> OK. Sometimes he even demands that they take
> him to the doctor to "prove" he's not sick.

Even though Malcolm's staying in conversations about his fear, he's working so hard to avoid the anxiety. Anxiety also causes some physical sensations, like headaches and stomachaches. Though I don't know anyone who likes feeling physically uncomfortable, if you're out of touch with your body, you might not even realize you've been avoiding situations that make you feel specific physical symptoms. If you're ignoring this valuable information, you might be accidentally causing yourself more discomfort in the long run.

There have likely been situations where you logically knew that avoiding something that wasn't truly dangerous made no sense, but you avoided it anyway. Anxiety tells you that facing your fear is not worth the risk. Bad things will happen, and you don't like bad things, do you? So you avoid *just in case*. This seems like a good idea, until the next time, when you again avoid, *just in case*. All those "just in cases" add up and get in the way of your life.

YOUR AVOIDANCE PROFILE

Everyone has their own avoidance profile, and understanding what you avoid, and when, can help you develop the tools to better manage your anxiety. Take some time to consider the following questions, and even write out your reflections if you'd like.

- **Do you avoid any specific external place or thing?** This can be a place like school or a specific restaurant. It can also be heights or closed spaces, needles and blood, specific foods, animals, or even being alone.

- **Do you avoid anything that causes specific physical sensations in your body?** For example, do you avoid drinking caffeine because it makes you jittery, or amusement park rides because you might get nauseous, or places where you might feel too warm or cold?

- **Do you avoid *thinking* about specific things because they make you uncomfortable?** This can include specific memories, or avoiding feeling uncomfortably sad.

- **Do you ask other people for reassurance that things are or will be OK?** Do you rely on others to face feared situations? This can include parents, teachers, or friends.

- **Do you do anything in your head to make yourself feel better when you're anxious?** For example:
  + Do you try to distract yourself from conversations that make you anxious?
  + Do you give yourself reassurance that things will be OK?
  + Do you mentally analyze events over and over to make sure they were OK?
  + Do you work through a mental checklist to convince yourself that there's nothing to be anxious about?
- **Do you check on things to get rid of your anxiety?** This can be things like locks, the stove, or where exits are in a room. It can also include checking if you did or did not write down specific things.
- **Do you feel the need to keep specific objects on you, just in case?** This can include things like medication that you don't need or antibacterial soap.

All the questions above point to patterns of avoidance. Some are more active, where you actually need to *do something* to avoid a feeling or situation—make a phone call, carry a medicine. Other avoidance patterns are more passive or mental—distraction and thought maneuvers count. The more you know about the way you avoid, the more you can do to combat these negative patterns.

FACING YOUR FEARS

Anxiety makes you avoid important situations out of fear. Exposure therapy is a technique designed to help you confront your fears through a series of doable steps. Facing your fears can teach you that the thing you're afraid of is not as dangerous as it seems and that you are able to cope with even the most unpleasant situations. Exposure has consistently been found to be the most effective way to treat a variety of anxiety problems, particularly phobias, obsessive-compulsive disorder (OCD), and panic attacks. It's also key in treating other disorders like social anxiety, separation anxiety, and generalized anxiety.

Doing exposure is like getting into a cold pool. You have two options: You can either jump right in, or you can gradually lower your body into the water inch by inch, first dipping a toe, then an ankle, and so on. Both ways will get you wet, eventually. Both ways will be uncomfortable (the pool is COLD!), but then your body will adjust to the temperature and you'll get used to it. There's no magic button to get you into the pool *and* have the water be warmer. You're going to have to experience some discomfort to swim.

Using exposure means breaking down feared situations and then doing them and seeing what happens. Sometimes you can do this in the real world. If you're afraid of heights, exposure might involve hanging out on a second-floor balcony for a while and tracking your fear, then moving to the third-floor balcony, and as you get comfortable, hanging out on higher and higher floors.

Know that the more you do something, the easier it is. The first time you hang out on the second floor, your anxiety might be an 8 on the 0 to 10 scale, but the sixty-fifth time you complete the same exposure, chances are your anxiety will not stay at that 8.

It is often easiest to do this by just going to high places, but sometimes you can use your imagination to do exposure as well. In these situations (called imaginal exposures), you might imagine going to high places instead of actually going to them, which can be helpful if you don't have access to tall buildings or if you're too nervous to start off with the real thing.

Know that fear doesn't go away overnight. Exposure sometimes works very quickly, but it can also take repeated sessions to see your gains, and it is often hard work. Just keep in mind that facing something you've been avoiding for a while is an accomplishment in its own right, and is a big deal.

FEAR LADDER

Facing fears is best done in small increments. You can break down your fear using something called a "fear ladder." You can use your avoidance profile answers from earlier in this chapter to identify where a fear ladder might help you face your fears. If you're avoiding things that you want or need to do, this is a good opportunity to tackle them. It could be learning a new skill, talking to specific people, raising your hand in class, doing your homework, or basically anything else. The more specific you can be in identifying the fear, the easier it will be to figure out exposure strategies. Here's how a fear ladder works:

1. **First think of the fear you want to overcome.** Focus on a situation where your avoidance has had a negative impact on your life. It should be something specific. For example, "I want to drive a car by myself." Your life is probably pretty difficult if you always avoid driving alone, so overcoming this fear would probably make your life easier.

2. **Set a specific goal.** Be very clear about what this goal will be. For example, "To drive by myself to Lee's house and back." When setting your goal, think not just about what you want to do but also when you want to do it (in the next week? month?) and how much or how often you want to do it.

3. **Break your goal down into four or more steps.** They should be steps that build on each other to get you to your goal. Rank each one from 0 to 10, with 10 being the most difficult and anxiety-provoking and 0 being not anxiety-provoking at all. The last step should match the specific goal you set at the beginning.

4. **For my driving example, steps might include:**

    + Sit in the driver's seat with the car on. (3/10)

    + Drive out of the driveway and around the block by myself. (6/10)

    + Drive a couple blocks and back by myself. (8/10)

    + Drive all the way to Lee's house by myself. (10/10)

    Try to be realistic about your ratings, and think about them as relative to each other. If driving long distances in a car is a 10, then backing out of the driveway is probably not also a 10.

5. **Try it out!** Anxiety during exposure practice is normal, but that anxiety is not dangerous. Start with the least anxiety-producing activity on your list and see what happens. If it seems too hard, brainstorm other steps that might be easier. If you succeed, be proud of your accomplishment! Give yourself a little reward before moving on to the next step. Feel proud that you took the first step in getting your life back from anxiety.

On the following page are some examples of fear ladders in action. Know that your fears are unique to you, so these fear hierarchies are not one-size-fits-all. These examples are to show you how the setup works.

FEAR: Petting or coming close to dogs

ACTIVITY	FEAR RANKING (0-10)
Pet a large dog off-leash	10
Pet a small dog off-leash	8
Pet a small dog on a leash	7
Walk past a dog park	6
Watch videos of large, aggressive-looking dogs	5
Watch a video of small dogs	4
Watch a dog through the window	3

FEAR: Speaking in social situations

ACTIVITY	FEAR RANKING (0-10)
Give a presentation in class	8
Ask a question in class	5
Say hi to someone I don't know in the hall	4
Ask a peer I don't know to borrow a pencil	6
Ask an adult where the bathroom is	3

TIPS FOR EXPOSURE SUCCESS

The best way to do exposure is to plan well. Good exposure is not "just" facing your fear; it's deciding to face your fear systematically. At their best, exposure exercises should work like shampoo directions: Rinse, lather, repeat. You plan an exercise, then try it out, debrief with yourself, and do it again. To do this well, it's important to know that you might be anxious when doing an exposure exercise. That's OK—your body is designed to have a fear reaction, and you're practicing to live your life better. Here are some tips to maximize your exposure exercises:

- **Plan in advance.** If stumbling into situations that you're afraid of made your fears go away, people wouldn't be afraid of much. Develop a solid exposure plan by referring to the fear ladder you created. Know what you're going in to do, and how long you're going to do it.

- **Take risks, but start small.** The most important part of doing exposure is sticking with it, so you don't need to start with the hardest thing on your list. Instead, start with something that you're willing to do no matter what, even if you *could* do something harder. If someone tells me they're afraid of the dark, but think they can stay in a dark room for 10 minutes a night,

I suggest they start with 5 minutes instead. To get started on the right foot, I'd rather focus on consistency instead of doing something hard only one time.

- **Reward yourself.** Exposure can be hard work! Choose something meaningful that you can do or give yourself for engaging in the exercise you chose. It can be a treat or an activity. Remember to reward yourself after you try the exercise, not before. Even if you feel like you've failed, reward yourself for trying. It's the attempts that are going to make the difference.

- **Change it up.** Vary the time and place. Research shows that variation makes you learn even better. Try the exercise at home, in school, after school—the more unpredictable, the better.

- **Keep track.** Track your anxiety in a journal before, during, and after the exercise. That way, you can track your progress over time.

- **It's OK to be anxious.** While you're completing an exercise, allow yourself to feel the fear if it's there and track it using the rating system. Staying in the fear will help you recognize that you *can* feel fear without it ruining your life.

EXPOSURE

USEFUL FOR: Getting rid of your anxious behaviors

TIME: Four times a week. Pick a new exercise weekly.

EQUIPMENT: Notebook or journal

Think of exposures as experiments: You're trying to determine whether the thing you're afraid of is actually true. To get to the answer, you need to identify what your core fear is. Ask yourself: What would happen if my fear came true? Maybe you'll be hurt, or embarrassed, or fail at something. Once you identify this core fear, write it down so you can look back after the exposure and determine if it came true.

Exposure can feel scary or hard, but it's important to stick with it. If you end up escaping or avoiding an exposure exercise, just "get back on the horse" and try again. It's perfectly OK to feel anxious during exposure—it's actually a signal that you're doing it right.

1. **Once you've set a specific goal, pick an activity on your fear ladder that you plan on practicing this week.** If you don't have a fear ladder yet, go back and make one.

2. **Before you do the exercises from your fear ladder, write down the following:**

   - What fears will you face with this first step on the ladder? What safety behaviors will you give up?
   - What do you fear most about this exercise? Be specific.
   - How long can you stick with this task? (For example, 10 minutes a day for a week.)

3. **Do the exercise from your fear ladder.**

   - Every five minutes, rate how anxious you're feeling on a scale of 0 to 10.
   - Also, pay attention to how much you want to run away or avoid the situation.
   - Describe your emotions to yourself while you're in the situation; for example, "I feel scared that . . ." Be specific.

4. **After you complete the exercise, ask yourself:**

   - How did it go? Did the thing you feared most come true?
   - Did you learn anything from this experience? Were you surprised by anything that happened?

- Is there anything you can do to vary up this experience next time? Remember that variety is good, so change up the time of day, the people you speak to, the type of dog you approach, or anything you can think of.

5. **Do each exposure exercise at least four times before you move on to the next activity.** The more exposure, the better, because it gives you more opportunity to learn. The more you do something, the easier and/or more rewarding it gets, so doing each step once is not enough. The more, the better.

TIP:

If you find yourself too overwhelmed to complete a step, though, you can go back to your fear ladder and choose a step that ranks lower on the anxiety scale, or create a half step. With this approach, you can work up to your goal in a realistic way.

IMAGINAL EXPOSURE

USEFUL FOR: Changing your response to your anxiety

TIME: Four times a day for a week

EQUIPMENT: Notebook journal

Your imagination is a very powerful tool. Sometimes you can imagine your way through your anxiety instead of facing it in real life. This can be helpful when you're not quite ready for real-life exposure. In this case, imaginal exposure is a warm-up or in-between step. It's also good for situations that don't occur very often in real life. If you're afraid of flying but have no travel plans anytime soon, this is an excellent tool. It's also good for situations in which you *can't* face your feared exposure in real life. If you're afraid of your house getting broken into while you sleep, we would not stage a break-in. Instead, use imaginal exposure.

When you're anxious about something that probably won't happen, like getting robbed or killed, the thoughts tend to pop up throughout your day. You end up playing a mental game of jack-in-the box, where you try to hold the terrifying thoughts down but then they keep popping back up. Imaginal exposure is a technique to take the power away from these thoughts by helping you recognize that you can think about even the most terrifying things, and that doesn't mean they will come true. In fact, our minds are programmed to get bored after facing something again and again!

~~~~~~~~~~~~~~~~~~~~~~~~~~~~

1. **Choose a fear you've identified as negatively impacting your life, but which you may not be ready or able to face in real life; for example, the fear of getting in a car crash.**

2. **Write out your "nightmare scenario" in the form of a short story.** Use your imagination to be as vivid as possible. Use all your senses to tell this story. What do you see? Hear? Smell? Taste? Touch? Imagine the details, including how your body feels in this feared situation and what thoughts you might have. Pretend that you're in this situation in real life, as if you were doing real exposure. Think about what you're afraid of and include that in your story. The aim here is to face your fear, so a good exposure story will make you feel afraid, and that's good.

3. **Once you've written out your story, read it over.** You can record yourself reading the story and listen to it if you prefer.

4. **After you've read or listened to your story:**

   • Rate how anxious you're feeling on a scale of 0 to 10.

   • Describe your current emotions about the situation; for example, "I feel scared that . . ." Be specific.

   • Did you learn anything from this experience? Were you surprised by anything that happened?

- Is there anything you can do to vary up this script next time? Can you make it more vivid?

5. **Read or listen to this story four times a day (it can be back-to-back; typically, these stories don't take very long to read).** Track your practice and your anxiety rating every day. Do they stay the same? Change?

TIP:

Facing your fears now can help you cope in the long term. So the more you can do to feel scared during this exercise, the better. You can combine imaginal and regular exposure exercises; for example, going to the top of a building and, while you're there, reading your script about your fear of falling off. As with all exposure exercises, do this several times. I know this skill seems counterintuitive, but facing feared situations takes away their power.

BODY EXPOSURE

USEFUL FOR: Challenging your beliefs about how dangerous physical symptoms are, especially during panic attacks

TIME: 5 minutes a day

EQUIPMENT: A small straw, an office chair

Remember that anxiety is made up of three parts—thoughts, behaviors, and sensations. The two previous exposure exercises targeted your behaviors. This exercise targets the physical sensations of anxiety. Body exposure lets you experience these "scary" anxiety sensations to see what happens. Know that some of these exercises will feel uncomfortable—that's the point! The point is to see whether your worst fears will come true if you bring on these symptoms on purpose. Will you pass out if you get too dizzy, or have a heart attack if you hyperventilate? This exposure will test it out.

On the following page is a list of exercises. It's a good idea to try them all to figure out which ones are most relevant to you. For each exercise, rate (1) how uncomfortable it makes you feel on a scale of 0 to 10, and (2) how anxious the sensation makes you feel on a scale of 0 to 10. Notice how each exercise feels, and describe to yourself how it is similar to your anxiety reaction. Repeat these exercises daily for a week, and compare your ratings. If there's a specific physical symptom of your anxiety that you fear, this is a chance to see if it's actually as dangerous as you think.

- **Straw breathing:** Using a small straw or stirrer, breathe in and out through the straw while holding your nose.
- **Spinning:** Sit in an office chair. Spin around as fast as you can for one minute.
- **Planking:** Hold a push-up position for one minute.
- **Shaking your head:** Shake your head from side to side for 30 seconds.
- **Running in place:** Run in place, or up and down steps, for one minute.
- **Holding your breath:** Hold your breath for 30 seconds.

TIP:

Be aware if avoidance creeps in. Remember that avoidance can be subtle, like stopping early or "cheating" on an exercise. You'll get the most benefit by fully engaging.

BREAKING BAD HABITS

Avoidance is not the only behavior pattern that keeps anxiety going. There are other types of bad habits that may create anxiety loops. When you engage in these negative patterns of thinking and feeling, you continue to feed your anxiety and panic. Read through the list of bad habits in this section. Do you see any of these behaviors in yourself? Are these habits things that you want to change? The first step is noticing your own behavior, so even being able to identify your actions is a good first step.

PERFECTIONISM

What's wrong with trying to be perfect? High standards can be a good thing—they help you become the best version of yourself, right? Perfectionism involves setting standards that are so high that they're almost impossible to meet. And if you're a perfectionist, chances are that you believe anything short of this (nearly impossible) goal is the same as failure.

Everyone makes mistakes sometimes. Most people don't enjoy making mistakes, but they can probably accept that they're part of life and work to learn from them. If you're a perfectionist, though, mistakes are a different story: They're a catastrophic sign that you've failed, and need to be avoided at all costs. Take Sarah, a straight-A student who believes that any grade less than perfect is basically a sign that she's less capable than others. She studies for hours to make sure she knows the material backward, forward, and upside down. She turns down social opportunities to study, because she's terrified to make mistakes. Even though her performance is excellent and her teachers only have amazing things to say about her, she's constantly stressed about her grades and worried about failure.

To ease the stress and anxiety that comes with trying to be perfect, there are a couple steps you can take:

1. **Work to identify your perfectionist tendencies.**

2. **What thought distortions are you using?** Check out "Analyzing Your Thoughts" (PAGE 98) and "Coping Statements" (PAGE 102) to figure out your patterns of thinking and to read some suggestions about how to change your thinking.

3. **Use exposure by designing a fear ladder for your perfectionism:** Mess stuff up on purpose, show up five minutes late for an appointment, or make a mistake on an assignment. Notice whether your worst fears come true, and if they do, can you cope?

RUMINATION

When you ruminate, you revisit negative experiences in your mind over and over. It may *feel* like it gets you closer to solving a problem or understanding the situation better, but it doesn't do either. Instead, rumination is closely associated with depression, and you end up in a continuous loop of negative thoughts.

You can get stuck ruminating about anything—that date you just went on, your upcoming soccer game, or a sore throat that you started to feel. The danger of rumination is that it can make you feel bad about yourself, or become a self-fulfilling prophecy when you get so stuck in it that it keeps you from your goals.

The problem with rumination is that telling yourself to stop thinking about whatever is bothering you only makes it worse. If I tell you not to think of pink elephants, you're bound to think of pink elephants. One of the best strategies for handling rumination is a combination of the mindfulness skills from Chapter 3 and the exposure techniques outlined at the beginning of this chapter. Bringing awareness to your thoughts without trying to control them might make you anxious. That's OK here. Focusing on that emotion is actually an exposure technique! You're facing the fear that you have instead of thinking through your problem and trying to solve it.

COMPULSIONS

Compulsions are behaviors you engage in to relieve your anxiety, particularly in obsessive-compulsive disorder (OCD). Think about it like this: Obsessions are your anxious thoughts. They're sticky and uncomfortable and lead to distress and anxiety. When you feel that anxiety, you want to *do something* to get rid of it. That thing you do is a compulsion. It reduces your anxiety and makes you feel better, but only in the short term.

In the long term, following through on compulsions actually makes you more obsessed. Here's how this looks:

> Keisha leaves the house and then worries that she might have left the door unlocked. She fears that if the door is unlocked, someone might get in and steal something. These thoughts make her anxious, so she goes back and checks to make sure the door is locked. When she checks the door, she feels better, but the feeling doesn't last. A few minutes later, the worried thoughts come back: "Should I have checked the windows? Maybe I left one unlocked. Or maybe I didn't turn the door lock all the way." The obvious solution is to repeat the compulsion, so Keisha goes back to check the windows and recheck the door lock, just in case.

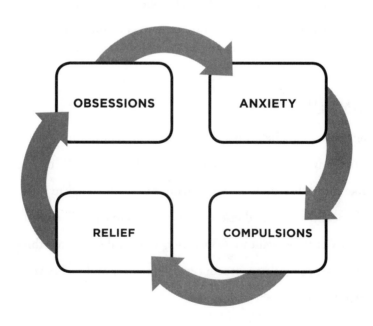

Research shows that the best way to stop the cycle of obsessions and compulsions is to cut out the compulsions completely. I know this sounds hard, and it might be, but it's worth it. Compulsions will never give you long-term relief. By not giving in to your compulsions in the short term, you may find that you can live with your anxiety, and that sometimes anxious thoughts even subside when they're not fed with compulsive behavior. To help get rid of your compulsions, you can use these strategies:

1. **Begin by tracking your compulsions.** Use the "Track Your Anxiety" method on PAGE 23.

2. **Design a fear ladder.** This should involve cutting out your compulsions and facing your obsessions.

3. **Pick one compulsion to target with exposure.** You can try cutting it out completely, but if that doesn't feel doable, think about ways to push it off. Tell yourself, "I won't check the locks until 9 p.m." Next week, make it 9:30 p.m.

WITHHOLDING EMOTIONS

Pushing away your uncomfortable emotions when they pop up *seems* like a good idea. After all, you might be holding this book precisely because anxiety is uncomfortable and hard to deal with. The problem is that feelings don't stay ignored.

Feelings work like soda bottles. If you shake one as hard as you can, and then open it, it *will* explode. Feelings eventually bubble over, and if you're suppressing them, they tend to explode in an unmanageable way. Instead, open that shaken soda bottle slowly to release the carbonation a little at a time until it's manageable. For emotions, this means feeling them when they come up. This helps you learn that you *can* handle them, even if they're uncomfortable.

Using mindfulness exercises can help you learn this approach to feeling emotions instead of avoiding them by staying with them in the moment and noticing them without judgment.

MUSCLE TENSION

The physical response to anxiety can be uncomfortable, feel stressful, and make you feel like you can't really relax your body. You hold on to your anxiety by keeping your muscles tense. This makes your body on edge, and basically primes you for more anxious thoughts and behaviors. Your body is ready to spring into anxiety mode at a moment's notice.

This muscle tension can hurt—have you ever noticed yourself grinding your teeth or clenching your fists when you're anxious? For some, this muscle tension happens all day long, just on a milder level. This can mean that you're even breathing more shallowly— when your stomach is tense, you tend to breathe from your chest instead of your whole belly, which makes you feel out of breath more quickly, and generally more light-headed.

If these symptoms sound familiar, you might be a person who carries your anxiety in your body.

Here are some strategies you can try:

- Focus on breathing skills, like color breathing (PAGE 55), square breathing (PAGE 64), or abdominal breathing (PAGE 83).
- Try progressive muscle relaxation (PAGE 50) or the body scan exercise (PAGE 57). Noticing the difference between tension and relaxation, and setting an alarm on your phone to go off every hour to check for tension in your muscles, is a good trick.

SUBSTANCE USE

If you use drugs, smoking, vaping, or alcohol to manage your anxiety, it can seem helpful. After all, you don't feel anxious when you're drunk, right? The problem is the rebound effects. When you use drugs or alcohol, you choose feeling good in the short term over feeling good in the long term. The only way around your anxiety is through it, and if you avoid feeling anxious, you're not going to learn the strategies to handle it when it does pop up.

Also, using substances to control your anxiety leaves you with fewer options when you can't use drugs or alcohol. Think about it like this: You're in an important class, and you get hit with a wave of anxiety. All you want to do is run out of the classroom, go to your car, and smoke to calm down, but you know you'll miss important material and possibly get in trouble.

There's another hidden issue too: Many of the substances can also make you more anxious. You might not realize it, but stimulants—caffeine, nicotine—bring on some of those physical symptoms of anxiety. They also can have addictive properties that make your life harder instead of easier.

Instead, try and identify the thoughts you have that make you want to turn to substances—use the method in "Monitor Your Thoughts, Feelings, and Behaviors" (PAGE 25) to figure out what your triggers are. That will point you in the right direction and help you identify different options when you want to turn to substances. You can also check out some of the skills in this chapter, especially "Opposite Action" on the following page, to try and replace any bad habits with a healthier one.

STOPPING UNWANTED BEHAVIORS

Do you recognize any of the above bad habits in yourself? Think about whether they cause any problems in your life. The skills on the following pages will help you challenge avoidance and unhealthy or unhelpful habits. You might have been engaging in negative behavior patterns for a while and gotten used to coping with anxiety a certain way, so changing your behavior can be hard (if it was easy, you would have done it already!). With practice, though, you can create new habits.

OPPOSITE ACTION

USEFUL FOR: Changing uncomfortable emotions

TIME: Once a day

Remember that all emotions are normal and have a purpose—to urge you into acting a certain way. Acting the opposite of how you feel seems totally counterintuitive, but it's a great strategy for resisting the pull of painful emotions. Your goal with this exercise is not to suppress your feelings; it's to act differently from how you feel. This is a good strategy for when your emotion doesn't fit the situation.

1. **Identify the emotion that you're feeling right now.** Are you feeling anxious, sad, angry, or something else?
2. **Think about how your emotion wants you to act right now; oftentimes this means:**

   - Anxiety usually makes you want to avoid or run away.
   - Anger usually makes you want to yell, scream, or attack.
   - Sadness usually makes you want to withdraw.

3. **Think about whether this action is warranted right now.** What would be the consequences of acting the way you feel in this situation?

4. **If the consequences are mainly negative, try acting exactly the opposite.** Teenagers are known to be rebellious, so channel that inner rebellion to do the opposite of what your emotion wants you to do. Continue this opposite action until you feel the negative emotion subside.

- If you're anxious, face that fear again and again.
- If you're angry, do something nice for the person you want to attack, or practice empathy toward them.
- If you're sad, engage in something active rather than withdraw.

> **TIP:**
>
> Acting the opposite of how your emotions want you to act is like using exposure to face your emotions—it might feel uncomfortable, since it challenges your habitual patterns. Before you give up, try it several times, say every day for a week, and see if it has any impact on your emotions. Opposite action is also a good strategy for managing the urge to use substances.

POSITIVE REINFORCEMENT

USEFUL FOR: Making a hard task easier

TIME: 10 minutes of planning, once a week

EQUIPMENT: Notebook or journal (optional)

Changing bad habits is a challenge. Rewards can keep you motivated to stay on track and make the changes you need to make for a healthier you. Little kids get stickers and small prizes for good work all the time, and guess what? The same trick works on adults! Everyone likes rewards. A teen once told me that she finds it really hard to face uncomfortable feelings, but that the task is easier when she has something to look forward to. We developed a rewards system that could keep her motivated through the rough patches by acknowledging even the small steps, and it worked fantastically!

1. **Think about activities you really enjoy or items you'd like to get yourself.** You may find it helpful to write them down. Consider small activities like playing Xbox or treating yourself to ice cream, or even small items you'd like to buy that are

within your budget. You can also include upcoming events or activities that you'd look forward to doing. You can go back to the "Plan Activities You Value" exercise on PAGE 78 to identify some pleasurable activities.

2. **Pick a weekly target that will earn you a reward when reached.** Focus on goals you can control, like practicing mindfulness three times a week, or facing a specific fear on your fear ladder, or tracking your thoughts four days a week. Choose targets that seem doable. You can always do more, but it's easy to get frustrated if you don't meet goals that were set too high.

3. **Identify a reward for meeting a specific goal.** Use the list you came up with above. When you meet that goal, treat yourself!

TIP:

Don't give yourself the reward until *after* you meet your target. You can also reward yourself for smaller targets or small steps that move you toward a larger goal. I use this all the time—for example, if I work for 30 minutes, I get to take a 5-minute Internet break.

COPING CARDS

USEFUL FOR: Identifying the coping skills that work for you

TIME: 20 minutes for setting them up. Use as needed.

EQUIPMENT: Index cards

One of the trickiest parts of using skills to manage anxiety is remembering what the skills are and how to use them. They will become second nature with practice, but until you get there, you can create a cheat sheet of the coping strategies that work for you by writing them down on index cards.

1. **Choose strategies from the list below, or any of the skills in this book, that you want to have on hand:**

   • A reminder that a physical symptom of anxiety, like shortness of breath or nausea, is just your fight-flight-freeze response. List skills that help you manage these symptoms, like deep breathing or exercise.
   • Your favorite mindfulness strategy, paired with the thoughts or behaviors it helps you manage.
   • A list of the thinking traps you habitually fall into, paired with a list of reality checks or coping statements.

- Positive coping statements to counter your negative self-talk, like "I can do this, even if it's hard!"
- A reminder that feelings fade; for example, "Anxiety is like a wave; it rises and falls. I can surf this wave." You can also recall the visualization exercises with phrases like "My thoughts are like a leaf in a river."
- A reminder of your goals for when exposure feels overwhelming: "I'm learning to be comfortable with being uncomfortable."

2. **Write the name of the strategy on one side of an index card.**
3. **On the other side, describe the strategy in detail.** Include other information you might find helpful for yourself. For example, "Use this when I need to calm down fast."
4. **Feel free to laminate the cards and put them on a ring to carry with you, or decorate them to fit your personality.**

TIP:

If you're not into carrying around cards, you can write down your strategies in the "Notes" app of your phone or snap pictures of your cards so you can look at them without being obvious. Whatever form you choose, sites like Pinterest and Instagram are great places to find positive coping statements.

PROBLEM-SOLVING

USEFUL FOR: Identifying solutions to problems

TIME: 5 to 10 minutes, as often as needed

EQUIPMENT: Notebook or journal (optional)

It's easy to get caught up in your anxiety and let your thoughts and behaviors snowball. This makes it hard to recognize when a problem has a solution. When something is stressing you out, focusing your mental energy on fixing the problem can relieve some of the tension.

1. **Identify the problem you're facing right now.** Try to be as clear and specific as possible. Only focus on one problem at a time.

2. **Break it down.** If the problem is big and broad, like "I'm not going to get all my work done," narrow it down to something specific, like "I have a four-page essay due on Tuesday, and I feel overwhelmed."

3. **Brainstorm possible solutions.** Remember, the rule for brainstorming is that there are no bad answers. Try to generate as many solutions as you can. For the four-page essay, you could

write an outline, e-mail a teacher to ask for an extension, blow off the paper completely, etc. Avoid evaluating the solutions at this point. Ask friends and family for help if you're having a hard time coming up with solutions.

4. **Evaluate your solutions.** Identify pros and cons for each one. Write these down if you want.

5. **Pick the best solution for you.** There will probably not be a perfect solution—it's just about what works right now. Choose an option that won't be too hard to try out, even if it's not your ideal.

TIP:

Problem-solving only works for problems with solutions. When your anxiety latches on to an irrational fear like "I'm afraid I'm going to have a heart attack in the middle of a basketball game," you're better off using other strategies instead.

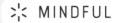
VISUALIZE SUCCESS

USEFUL FOR: Focusing on your success

TIME: 5 minutes, three times a week

EQUIPMENT: Notebook or journal

Think about how much mental energy you spend living with anxiety. If you're afraid of flying, you've probably spent a lot of time thinking about all the different ways a flight could go wrong. On the flip side, how much time have you spent thinking about what effectively managing your anxiety would look like? Visualization can help you imagine a successful outcome. Athletes use this technique to mentally rehearse successfully passing a ball or making a shot.

1. **Think about a specific anxiety-inducing situation you're facing, like staying home alone, speaking to a new classmate, performing well on an exam, or going to the doctor.**

2. **Take a few minutes to write out what a successful outcome would be like.** Get specific and use all your senses. What would success visually look like? How would it feel in your body? (Remember that anxiety often comes with physical discomfort, so it might be unrealistic to expect your body to be calm while killing a spider.) What sounds would you hear?

(Cheering? Applause?) What would others say to you, or what would you say to yourself? And remember that you're still you, so aim for realistic—not ideal—success.

3. **After you've given this scenario some thought, lie down comfortably.** Close your eyes and bring your attention to your breath. Breathe in and out deeply and follow each inhale and exhale.

4. **Now turn your attention to your imagined success scenario.** Visualize yourself completing the task you've written about. Imagine the sights, sounds, and physical sensations. Imagine what you would say or do.

TIP:

Practice this skill before entering a situation that makes you anxious. Once you're actually in the anxiety-provoking situation, use exposure and mindfulness techniques to get you across the finish line.

FEELINGS MEDITATION

USEFUL FOR: Feeling less overwhelmed

TIME: 10 minutes

When you experience a lot of anxious self-talk, you may feel overwhelmed and down on yourself. This meditation can help you release some of these worried thoughts.

1. **Find a quiet place to sit or lie down.** Close your eyes and get into a comfortable position.
2. **Use your breath to anchor yourself in the present moment.** Mindfully notice yourself inhale, then exhale. Your anxious thoughts may swirl around your brain. Notice that distraction and gently return your attention to your breath.
3. **As you breathe in, imagine inhaling all the calm that you have.** As you breathe out, exhale all your stress, negativity, and overwhelming thoughts.

4. **As you breathe in again, imagine inhaling all your coping thoughts.** As you breathe out, imagine exhaling all your negativity. Feel it leaving your body.

5. **Continue using your breath as an anchor.** Breathe in strength, positivity, and healthy thoughts. Breathe out your irrational beliefs, worries, anxieties, and pain.

PANIC ATTACKS

A panic attack is the physical manifestation of anxiety. Chapter 1 described the three parts of anxiety (and all other emotions): thoughts, physical sensations, and behaviors. Like all emotional reactions, a panic attack involves all three parts in a very specific way. Let's break it down:

- **The physical sensations:** This is the key element of a panic attack, because your body goes into full fight-flight-freeze mode. These physical symptoms of anxiety tend to intensify quickly in a few minutes. You might notice some of the symptoms detailed on the following page.

- **The thoughts:** When your body has a fight-flight-freeze response, your natural instinct is to prepare for danger. When you have a panic attack, you prepare for danger but find none, so you then focus attention on your physical symptoms. Common thoughts during a panic attack are:
  + "I must be going crazy."
  + "I'm going to lose control."
  + "I'm going to have a heart attack."
  + "I'm going to die."

SYMPTOMS OF A PANIC ATTACK

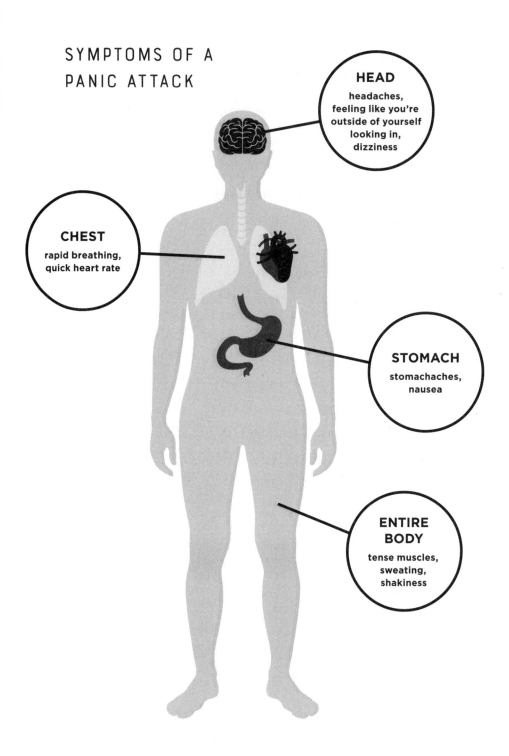

HEAD
headaches, feeling like you're outside of yourself looking in, dizziness

CHEST
rapid breathing, quick heart rate

STOMACH
stomachaches, nausea

ENTIRE BODY
tense muscles, sweating, shakiness

- **The behaviors:** When you feel this extreme physical discomfort and have such scary thoughts, it's only natural to want to escape. You might run out of the room for some fresh air or begin avoiding situations in which you previously had a panic attack. You might begin relying on safety signals, like calling your parents or carrying around a specific item.

One of the hallmarks of a panic attack is the feeling that they come "out of the blue." This can feel incredibly scary and dangerous, especially the first time. In reality, though, panic works like any other type of negative emotion. There's always a trigger, and that trigger can be a thought, a physical sensation, or a behavior. Panic gets you stuck in the cycle of anxiety. Once you begin obsessing about a physical symptom, you'll likely find one. When you escape or avoid the situation once, you think, "Wow, I got out right in time. Otherwise my fear would have come true!" So you keep avoiding and escaping. The main difference is that the symptoms of panic attacks are mostly physical, and individuals who experience them are more likely to believe that these bodily symptoms are dangerous.

This is an example of how the panic cycle works:

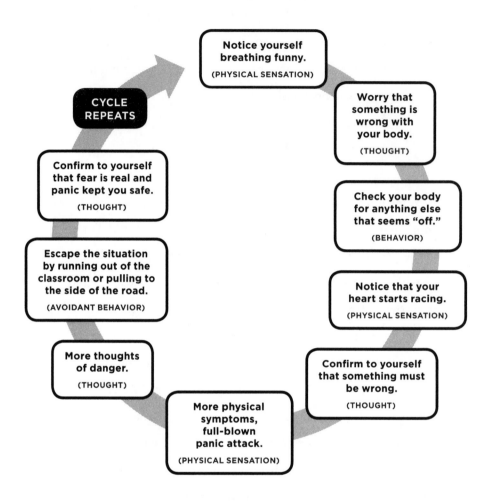

Notice yourself breathing funny.
(PHYSICAL SENSATION)

Worry that something is wrong with your body.
(THOUGHT)

Check your body for anything else that seems "off."
(BEHAVIOR)

Notice that your heart starts racing.
(PHYSICAL SENSATION)

Confirm to yourself that something must be wrong.
(THOUGHT)

More physical symptoms, full-blown panic attack.
(PHYSICAL SENSATION)

More thoughts of danger.
(THOUGHT)

Escape the situation by running out of the classroom or pulling to the side of the road.
(AVOIDANT BEHAVIOR)

Confirm to yourself that fear is real and panic kept you safe.
(THOUGHT)

CYCLE REPEATS

EARLY WARNING SIGNS

With practice, you can begin to recognize early warning signs for panic attacks. These signs are specific to your experience, so you can understand them better by keeping track of them. Learn the unique fingerprint of thoughts, sensations, and behaviors by writing them down as soon as they happen. Notice which symptoms come first and the situations in which they are triggered. For some people, a trigger will be a physical symptom. For others, it will be a thought.

> When Sima was having panic attacks, she came in for therapy. We began tracking her panic, and she realized she always panicked in math class. She was surprised that her symptoms always began with a specific thought: "I can't escape if I need to." Then she would feel itchy, and more uncomfortable thoughts and sensations would follow. Once she identified this pattern, she was able to use exposure techniques to stay in the situation instead of escaping. She realized that when she did so, the panic symptoms went away on their own.

While noticing early warning signs is a healthy way to begin managing panic attacks, the goal is *not* to resist or escape the sensations or thoughts that arise. This actually makes the panic stronger. Instead, when you notice symptoms of a panic attack, simply let yourself be aware of what is happening. Then grab a pen and rate the symptoms on a scale of 0 to 10, with 10 being the worst. Ask yourself, "Can I manage this *right now*?" instead of spiraling into anxious thinking about what it could be. Wait five minutes and notice if anything changes.

THE TRUTH ABOUT PANIC ATTACKS

Here's a secret about panic attacks: They're not dangerous. While they can be incredibly scary, they're just a false alarm trying to convince you to respond to imaginary danger. When you feel one coming on, remind yourself of these truths:

- **A PANIC ATTACK IS NOT A HEART ATTACK.** People who have panic attacks might end up at the doctor or in the emergency room. The symptoms *feel* medically dangerous, but in reality, they're not. Once a doctor clears you, there's no reason to fear that panic will turn into a heart attack or any other life-threatening illness.

- **A PANIC ATTACK WILL NOT MAKE YOU SUFFOCATE.** During a panic attack, you actually breathe in *more* oxygen. It might feel like you're having trouble breathing because you're hyper-ventilating—breathing so quickly that it makes you dizzy or light-headed. This feels uncomfortable because you're breathing in oxygen more quickly than you're breathing out carbon dioxide. It might feel like suffocation, but it is not.

- **A PANIC ATTACK WILL NOT MAKE YOU LOSE CONTROL.** Anxiety wants you to think that you might lose control or go crazy if you don't follow your fight-flight-freeze instinct. The truth is that when you're panicking, you're actually in control—that's what makes you engage in avoidant behaviors like running away. You might feel like you got to safety "just in time," but that feeling of safety is just another way your anxiety is trying to trick you.

- **A PANIC ATTACK ALWAYS HAS A TRIGGER.** Panic attacks can feel totally random, but there's always a trigger, even if you can't identify one in the moment. Once you've become more aware of your triggers, panic attacks will be easier to manage.

COPING WITH PANIC ATTACKS

The absolute best way to manage and stop panic attacks is to embrace them. I know that sounds ridiculous, but the more you face them, the more you'll see that they're not really as dangerous as you fear. Most importantly, you'll see that you are able to cope. Once your brain gets that message, the panic attacks will go away (or at least lessen in intensity) because you've broken the anxiety cycle. This exercise offers a step-by-step approach to handling your panic attacks.

1. **Keep track!** Use the "Track Your Anxiety" exercise (PAGE 23) to identify your triggers or the panic-inducing situation. Remember to note your thoughts, physical sensations, and behaviors.

2. **Identify your thinking traps.** Catastrophizing and jumping to conclusions are the two typical thinking errors people make when they're panicking. Refer to the "Label It" exercise (PAGE 99) to identify your own thinking errors, and reality-check yourself using the "Examine the Evidence" (PAGE 100) and "Coping Statements" (PAGE 102) skills.

3. **Be aware that it's hard to use thinking skills *during* a panic attack.** Once you're in panic mode, logic tends to fly out of the window because your body feels so uncomfortable. So use these skills before or after a panic attack hits.

4. **One way to manage panic attacks is through exposure.** Come up with a panic fear ladder (PAGE 123) by identifying five panic-inducing things you've been avoiding. Then commit to staying in one of these situations for a given length of time, *no matter what*. For example, "I'll stay in the car for five minutes, even if I start feeling panicky."

5. **Use body exposure.** Do the exercises listed on PAGE 135, and notice if any of them resemble your panic attack symptoms. If some of these exercises make you anxious, you can add them to your panic fear ladder.

6. **During a panic attack, use any mindfulness exercise you like to stay in the present moment, and with your thoughts and physical sensations.** Remember that you are stronger than you think you are.

If you're having trouble managing panic attacks on your own, or if you find that this book is not enough to help you change your relationship with anxiety, know that you still have options. Working one-on-one with a cognitive behavioral therapist can be a good way of figuring out which skills work for you.

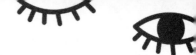

CONCLUSION

Living perfectly is an impossible goal. You're human and will experience normal human emotions, including anxiety, and some days will be better than others. Hopefully this book has showed you a different way of relating with your anxiety so you are better able to manage it as it arises, and bounce back a little faster when the days do get bad. As uncomfortable as it might feel sometimes (both physically and emotionally), your anxiety is part of who you are. So don't try to avoid, erase, or escape it. Your goal is to be more self-aware and accepting of difficult emotions. Only in this way can you see that just like those leaves on the river, even the most negative feelings eventually pass.

Remember that no single strategy will work for everyone. This book has presented a variety of tools and exercises so you can turn to different ones in different anxiety-inducing situations. If you're not sure which skills to use when, check out the Appendix on PAGE 168, where I lay out some "action plans" you can use to give yourself some structure. And if you're curious about learning more skills or getting more tips for managing anxiety, the Resources section on PAGE 171 lists suggestions for further reading, useful phone apps, and informative websites.

Know that progress hardly ever moves in a straight line. Even if you're committed to overcoming your anxiety, you might find yourself falling back into old habits sometimes. That's OK. You can always reread sections of this book that you found helpful and continue using the techniques you've learned. I know it's a downer to tell you that you're probably going to fail at some point, but everyone fails. Just be kind to yourself, keep practicing, and celebrate even the small steps!

APPENDIX

ACTION PLANS

The best way to use this book is to commit to a plan of action. Plans don't need to be elaborate to be effective. This is an opportunity to manage stress, not create more! Even if you feel ready for more, try to avoid packing too much in at once. Many of these strategies need time to become habits, and taking a step-by-step approach is the best way to make these new skills a part of your routine.

Below are some sample programs. Feel free to follow these or create your own. The idea is to slowly build yourself a toolkit of various coping skills you can use together or separately at different moments. To do this, practice each skill on its own for a week. Add a new skill the following week, and then practice the new one and the old one together. For example, start with tracking for a week. Then introduce a mindfulness exercise the second week, a healthy thinking exercise the third week, and so on. It typically takes between six weeks and six months to build up to a full anxiety management program.

Note that "Track Your Anxiety" (PAGE 23) and "Monitor Your Thoughts, Feelings, and Behaviors" (PAGE 25) are the foundation of any anxiety plan. You can't manage what you can't name. Use these steps to become more aware of your anxiety.

GENERALIZED ANXIETY

- Develop a self-care routine: Set up a regular bedtime, and aim to exercise for at least 30 minutes three times a week.
- Pick a mindfulness exercise to practice daily. If you're having trouble sleeping, try it before bed.

- Practice healthy thinking skills twice a week by labeling any thinking traps and identifying coping thoughts.
- Use opposite action daily for anxiety-provoking situations.
- Identify opportunities to do exposure once a week.
- Identify your go-to coping strategy. For example, carry around coping cards.

SOCIAL ANXIETY & SEPARATION ANXIETY

- Practice your go-to strategy for managing your negative thoughts four times a week.
- Practice mindfulness three times a week to reduce your baseline anxiety levels.
- Find pleasurable activities that you can engage in while you're in a social situation that makes you anxious. For example, if you're afraid of hanging out with large groups but you love ice-skating, skate in a crowd.
- Use exposure exercises to face a feared situation every day.
- Identify your go-to coping strategy. For example, carry around coping cards.

PHOBIAS

- Identify your thinking traps and coping statements you can use to face your phobia.
- Focus on exposure strategies by developing a fear ladder. The more often you can face your fear, the better. You can gradually build up to your core fear, or do longer exposure sessions to see quicker results.
- Identify the coping strategies that work for you in the moment when you feel anxious.

PANIC ATTACKS

- Use the "Coping with Panic Attacks" plan on PAGE 164.
- Practice mindfulness five times a week to reduce your baseline levels of anxiety.
- Make sure to focus on your own self-care. Think about your sleep, diet, and exercise routine. This is especially true for calming physical symptoms.
- Engage in activities you value three times a week to reduce your baseline anxiety.

OBSESSIVE-COMPULSIVE DISORDER (OCD)

- Track your obsessive anxious thoughts and compulsions (PAGE 23) daily for a week.
- Use this tracking information to create a fear ladder for your compulsions.
- Identify your thinking traps and come up with coping statements for them that you can use twice a week.
- The best treatment for OCD is exposure, exposure, exposure! Do exposure exercises every day. Use your fear ladder.
- Develop a self-care routine that includes pleasurable activities and exercise.
- Stress makes OCD symptoms worse, so find a mindfulness exercise that works for you and practice it five times a week.
- Identify your go-to coping strategy. For example, carry around coping cards.

RESOURCES

APPS (AVAILABLE FOR IOS AND ANDROID)

- Calm
- Headspace
- MindShift CBT
- Smiling Mind
- Stop, Breathe and Think
- Take a Chill (iOS only)

WEBSITES

www.abct.org

Visit the Association for Behavioral and Cognitive Therapy (ABCT) website for information about CBT. They also have a therapist directory to help you find a CBT therapist near you.

www.adaa.org

Anxiety Disorders Association of America has resources to help you understand anxiety and how to find a therapist.

www.anxietycanada.com

Anxiety Canada has resources and worksheets for managing anxiety.

www.self-compassion.org

Dr. Kristen Neff's website has resources on building self-compassion.

www.sleepfoundation.org

Visit the National Sleep Foundation's website for information about healthy sleep habits.

www.trailstowellness.org

The Trails to Wellness website has information, videos, and handouts on CBT for teens.

www.youtube.com/thepsychshow

"The Psych Show" with Dr. Ali Mattu is a series of short videos on mental health and CBT information.

BOOKS

Cognitive Behavioral Therapy Made Simple: 10 Strategies for Managing Anxiety, Depression, Anger, Panic, and Worry, by Seth J. Gillihan

Conquer Negative Thinking for Teens: A Workbook to Break the Nine Thought Habits That Are Holding You Back, by Mary Karapetian Alvord and Anne McGrath

Mindfulness for Teen Anxiety: A Workbook for Overcoming Anxiety at Home, at School, and Everywhere Else, by Christopher Willard

Talking Back to OCD, by John S. March with Christine M. Benton

The Self Compassion Workbook for Teens: Mindfulness and Compassion Skills to Overcome Self-Criticism and Embrace Who You Are, by Karen Bluth

FOR PARENTS:

Helping Your Anxious Child: A Step-by-Step Guide for Parents, by Ronald Rapee et al.

You and Your Anxious Child: Free Your Child from Fears and Worries and Create a Joyful Family Life, by Anne Marie Albano with Leslie Pepper

REFERENCES

American Academy of Sleep Medicine. "Recommended Amount of Sleep for Pediatric Populations: A Consensus Statement of the American Academy of Sleep Medicine." Accessed January 6, 2020. **https://jcsm.aasm.org/doi/10.5664/jcsm.5866**.

Anxiety Disorders Association of America. "Understand the Facts." Accessed January 6, 2020. **https://adaa.org/understanding-anxiety**.

Association for Behavioral and Cognitive Therapies. "Get Information" main page. Accessed January 6, 2020. **www.abct.org/Information**.

Birmaher, Boris, et al. "Screen for Child Anxiety Related Disorders (SCARED)." Accessed January 6, 2020. **www.midss.org/sites/default/files/scaredchild1.pdf**.

Ehrenreich-May, Jill, et al. *Unified Protocols for Transdiagnostic Treatment of Emotional Disorders in Children and Adolescents: Therapist Guide*. New York: Oxford University Press, 2018.

Harm Research Institute. "Sheehan Scales and Structured Diagnostic Interviews: MINI (Mini International Neuropsychiatric Interview)." Accessed January 6, 2020. **https://harmresearch.org/index.php/about-us/david-v-sheehan-md-mba/sheehan-scales-and-structured-diagnostic-interviews**.

National Institute of Mental Health. "Ask Suicide-Screening Questions (ASQ) Toolkit." Accessed January 6, 2020. **www.nimh.nih.gov/research/research-conducted-at-nimh/asq-toolkit-materials**.

National Sleep Foundation. "Sleep Topics." Accessed January 6, 2020. **www.sleepfoundation.org/sleep-topics**.

Neff, Kristin. "Self-Compassion Guided Meditations and Exercises." Accessed January 6, 2020. **https://self-compassion.org/category/exercises**.

Trails to Wellness. "Materials." Accessed January 6, 2020. **https://trailstowellness.org/materials**.

Willard, Christopher. *Mindfulness for Teen Anxiety*: *A Workbook for Overcoming Anxiety at Home, at School, and Everywhere Else*. Oakland, CA: Instant Help Books, 2014.

EXERCISE/SKILL INDEX

FOCUS

Anxiety Quiz, 7–9

Are You Getting Enough Sleep, 34

Find the Root of Your Anger, 69–70

Monitor Your Thoughts, Feelings, and Behaviors, 25–26

Short- and Long-Term Consequences, 27–28

Track Your Anxiety, 23–24

Visualize the New You, 29–30

Your Avoidance Profile, 120–121

MINDFUL

Abdominal Breathing, 83–84

Be Kind to Yourself, 87–88

Be Your Own Friend, 109–110

Body Scan, 57–59

Color Breathing, 55–56

Do One Thing at a Time, 44–45

Feelings Meditation, 155–156

Five Senses Activity, or 5-4-3-2-1, 53–54

Lake Meditation, 46–47

Listen to Your Emotions, 81–82

Mindful Eating, 48–49

Progressive Muscle Relaxation, 50–52

Self-Soothing, 80

Settling Your Mind, 62–63

Sing Your Thoughts, 108

Square Breathing, 64–65

Thoughts on a River, 111–112

Visualization: Thoughts on a Train, 60–61

Visualize Success, 153–154

ACTION

Analyzing Your Thoughts, 98–101

Body Exposure, 135–136

Bully in a Playground, 113–114

Coping Cards, 149–150

Coping with Panic Attacks, 164–165

Coping Statements, 102–103

Exposure, 129–131

Imaginal Exposure, 132–134

Opposite Action, 145–146

Plan Activities You Value, 78–79

Positive Reinforcement, 147–148

Problem-Solving, 151–152

Realistic Thoughts, 106–107

Set Small Goals, 75–77

Worry Time, 104–105

Write It Out, 85–86

INDEX

A

Abdominal breathing, 83–84

    combining with visualization, 55

    in muscle tension, 143

Acceptance strategies, 13

Accepting your thoughts, 89–90

Action plans, 168–170

    for generalized anxiety, 168–169

    for obsessive-compulsive disorders, 170

    for panic attacks, 170

    for phobias, 169

    for separation anxiety, 169

    for social anxiety, 169

Actions, connecting emotions with, 72–73

Activities

    planning valued, 78–79, 148

    self-care, 3, 75–76, 170

Adaptive

    anger as, 67–68

    anxiety as, 14–15

Addiction, 13

Advance planning, 127

Agoraphobia, 7, 11

Anger, 13, 66

    abdominal breathing in reducing, 83–84

    as adaptive, 67

    dealing with, 67–68

    defined, 69

    as normal, 68

    roots of, 69–70

    triggers of, 19, 68, 69, 70

    writing in reducing your, 85–86

Anxieties

    as adaptive, 14–15

    avoidance and, 18–19

    benefits of, 6

    body scan in managing symptoms of, 57–59

    coping with, 3

    exposure in treating, 125, 129–131

    in families, 6

    forms of, 10–12

    generalized, 7, 10

    imaginal exposure and, 132–134

    imaging yourself without, 29–30

    managing, 1

    need for extra support, 20

    ok for, 128

    origin of, 6

    physical components of, 31

    ranking of, 24

    rebound effects of, 117

separating yourself from
thoughts, 111–114

separation, 8, 10

social, 8, 10

staying on track, 21–22

taking power away from
thoughts, 108

tracking, 23–24, 164, 170

triggers for, 15–16, 19

Automatic thoughts, being aware
of, 97

Avoidance, 115–118

anxiety and, 18–19

appearance of, 118–119

profile of, 120–121

reducing, as goal in CBT, 116

Awareness, nonjudgmental, 62–63

B

Bedtime

creating a relaxing ritual, 36

making a technology-free zone,
35

Behaviors, 15, 16

challenging your, 115–165

long-term consequences of,
27, 28

managing your, 1

monitoring, 25–26, 168

in panic attacks, 159

short-term consequences of,
27, 28

stopping unwanted, 144

Black-and-white thinking, 92

Body

moving your, 37–38

taking care of your, 31–32

Body exposure, 135–136, 165

holding your breath, 136

managing panic attacks
through, 165

planking in, 136

running in place, 136

shaking your head in, 136

spinning in, 136

straw breathing in, 136

Body scan, 57–59

in managing anxieties, 57–59

in muscle tension, 143

Brain, retraining your, 5–30

Brainstorming, 151–152

Breathing

abdominal, 55, 83–84, 143

color, 55–56, 143

square, 64–65, 143

in teaching mindfulness, 40

Bullying, 113–114

C

Caffeine, avoiding, 36

Catastrophizing, 93, 164

CBT for Insomnia (CBT-1), 36

Changing it up, 128

Chronic pain, 13

Cognitive behavioral therapy (CBT), 1, 5
    defined, 12
    effectiveness of, 13–14
    as model of emotions, 15–18
    reducing avoidance as goal in, 116
Color breathing, 55–56
    in muscle tension, 143
Compassion, finding for self, 109–110
Compulsions, 12, 139–141
    fear ladder in eliminating, 141
    targeting with exposure, 141
Conclusions, jumping to, 92–93, 101, 164
Coping cards, 149–150, 170
Coping statements, 102–103, 138
Coping strategies, identifying, 170
Couch to 5k app, 38

D

Depression, 13, 66
    dealing with, 71–73
    exercise and, 76–77
    reversal of cycle of withdrawal, 78
    suicidal thoughts as symptom of, 73
    turning of sadness into, 71
Description in mindfulness, 81
Discounting the positive, 94
Dogs, fear of petting or coming close to, 126

E

Eating, mindful, 48–49
Eating disorders, 13
Emotional reading, 93–94
Emotions, 66–88
    CBT model of, 15–18
    changing uncomfortable, 145–146
    connection with actions, 72–73
    defined, 66–67
    kindness in challenging, 87–88
    listening to, 81–82
    negative, 66
    setting goals with, 75–77
    sitting with your, 73–74
    withholding, 141–142
Escape, 115–118
Everyday relaxation, square breathing for, 64–65
Exercise
    depression and, 76–77
    effect on mood, 31
    need for regular, 36, 37–38
    phone apps for, 38
Exposure
    anxieties during, 125
    body, 135–136, 165
    changing up, 128
    in facing fears, 172
    in getting rid of anxious behaviors, 122–123, 129–131
    identifying opportunities for doing, 170
    imaginal, 123, 132–134

managing panic attacks through, 165

planning in advance, 127

rewarding yourself, 128

taking risks in, 127–128

targeting compulsions with, 141

tips for success in, 127–128

tracking in, 128

in treating anxieties, 122–123, 125, 129–131

in treating obsessive-compulsive behavior, 170

External environment, focusing attention on, 53

External triggers, 19

F

Families, anxieties in, 6

Fear ladder, 123–126, 130–131

in cutting out compulsions, 141

exposure in designing for perfectionism, 138

tracking information in creating, 170

Fears, 1

benefits of, 1

effects of, 1

facing your, 122–123

petting or coming close to dogs, 126

speaking in social situations, 126

as survival mechanism, 6

Feelings

meditation for, 155–156

monitoring, 25–26, 168

Fight, flight, or freeze, 6

Fortune-telling, 93

Friend

being your own, 109–110

exercising with a, 37

G

Generalized anxiety, 7, 10

action plans for, 168–170

Goals

breaking down into steps, 124

identifying rewards for meeting specific, 148

in overcoming fears, 124

setting small, 75–77

setting specific, 124, 129

Good, ignoring the, 94, 99

Grounding exercises, 53

H

Habits, breaking bad, 137–144

Hearing, in self-soothing, 80

Holding your breath in body exposure, 136

Hyperventilation, 162

I

Imaginal exposures, 123, 132–134

Index cards, for making coping cards, 149–150

Inner rebellion, 146

Insomnia, 32–33

Internal anxiety, coping with, 53

Internal triggers, 19

J

Journals

    coping statements in, 102–103

    imaginal exposures in, 132–134

    obstacles in, 29

    positive reinforcement and,
        147–148

    in problem-solving, 151–152

    tracking anxiety in, 128

    tracking your sleep in, 33

    visualization of success in,
        153–154

    visualizations in, 29

    worried thoughts in, 104–105

Judgment, holding off, 41

Jumping to conclusions, 92–93, 164

K

Kindness in challenging emotions,
    87–88

L

Labeling, 99, 164

Lake meditation, 46–47

Life stressors, 32

Listening to emotions, 81–82

Long-term consequences of
    behaviors, 27, 28

M

Magnification, 94

Meditation, 36

    feelings, 155–156

    lake, 46–47

    in teaching mindfulness, 40

Mental distraction, 117

Mental reassurance, 117

Mental review, 117

Mind-body connection, 31–65

Mindful eating, 48–49

Mindfulness, 1, 5, 19

    basics of, 40–41

    building into day, 44–45

    consistency in, 43

    defined, 12, 40

    description in, 81

    managing panic attacks
        through, 165

    observation in, 81

    openness in, 43

    practicing daily, 170

    preparing for, 42–43

    repetition in, 42

    research on, 39

    schedule for, 42

    senses in coping with, 53–54

    space for, 42

    staying in the present with,
        38–39

    time for, 42

    timing of, 36

    tracking, 43

Mind reading, 92

Mood, effects on, 31

Muscle tension, 142–143

N

Negative thinking, 109

changing, 95–96

zooming in on, 94

"No glow rule," 35

Nonjudgmental awareness, 62–63

Notebooks. See Journals

Nutrition, effect on mood, 31

O

Observations in mindfulness, 81

Obsessions, 139

Obsessive-compulsive disorders
(OCDs), 9, 11–12, 122, 139

action plans for, 170

exposure in treating, 122, 170

thinking traps in, 170

P

Panic attacks, 9, 11, 122, 157–163

action plans for, 170

behaviors in, 159

body exposure in, 135–136

coping with, 164–165

exposure in treating, 122

heart attacks and, 162

loss of control in, 163

physical sensations in, 157

suffocation and, 162

symptoms of, 158

thinking skills in, 165

thoughts in, 157

triggers for, 163

warning signs for, 160–161

Perfectionism, 137–138

Phobias, 8, 122

action plans for, 170

exposure in treating, 122

thinking traps in, 169

types of, 11

Phone apps for exercise, 38

Physical reactions, managing your, 1

Physical sensations, 15, 16, 25–26

in panic attacks, 157

Planking in body exposure, 136

Positive change

obstacles to making a, 30

self-awareness in making a, 5

Positive reinforcement, 147–148

Power, taking away from anxious
thoughts, 108

Practice, recognizing need for, 22

Problem-solving, journals in, 151–152

Procrastination, long-term
consequences of, 27, 28

Progressive muscle relaxation,
50–52

in muscle tension, 143

timing of, 36

R

Realistic thoughts, 89, 106–107

Reality-checking of worried
thoughts, 106–107
Rebound effects
of anxiety, 117
substance use and, 143
Reinforcement, positive, 147–148
Rewarding yourself, 128, 148
Risk taking, 127–128
Rumination, 138–139
Running away as manifestation of
avoidance, 118–119
Running in place, in body exposure,
136

S
Sadness, 66
dealing with, 71–73
as persistent, 71
turning into depression, 71
Safety, problems with seeking, 117
Self, finding compassion for, 109–
110
Self-awareness, in making a positive
change, 5
Self-care, 3, 75–76, 168, 171
Self-esteem, impact of negative
self-talk on, 109
Self-soothing, 80
Senses in coping with mindfulness,
53–54
Separation anxiety, 8, 10
action plans for, 169
7-Minute Workout app, 38

Shaking your head in body
exposure, 136
Short-term consequences of
behaviors, 27, 28
"Should" statements, 94–95
Skills, learning new, 22
Skin picking, 13
Sleep, 13
effect on mood, 31
falling faster, 35–36
importance of getting night's,
32–33, 34
quality of, 33
Sleep hygiene, 34
Sleep rhythms, shifts in, 33
Sleep schedule, need for, 35
Smell in self-soothing, 80
Snow globes in nonjudgmental
awareness, 62–63
Social anxiety, 8, 10
action plans for, 168–169
Social situations, fear of speaking
in, 126
Spinning, in body exposure, 136
Square breathing, 64–65
in muscle tension, 143
Square breathing for everyday
relaxation, 64–65
Statements
coping, 102–103, 138
creating summary, 107
"should," 94–95
Sticky mind, 90–91

Straw breathing, in body exposure, 136

Stress

abdominal breathing in reducing, 83–84

defined, 32

effect on mood, 31

Stress relief

color breathing in, 55–56

lake meditation in, 46–47

Substance use, 143–144

Success, visualization of, 153–154

Suicidal thoughts, 73

Summary statements, creating, 107

Support, asking for, 21

T

Taste in self-soothing, 80

Therapist, finding a, 20, 73

Thinking. See also Thoughts

black-and-white, 92

coping statements in developing healthy, 102–103

healthy skills in, 97

negative, 109

Thinking skills

in labeling generalized anxiety, 168–169

during panic attacks, 165

Thinking traps, 91–95

all or nothing as, 92

catastrophizing as, 93, 164

emotional reasoning as, 93–94

identifying, 106, 164

ignoring the good as, 94

jumping to conclusions as, 92–93, 164

in obsessive-compulsive disorder, 170

in phobias, 169

"should" statements as, 94–95

Thoughts, 15, 16. See also Thinking

accepting your, 89–90

analyzing, 98–101

changing your, 89–114

distortions of, in perfectionism, 138

evaluating, 100

identifying, 98–99

labeling, 99

limiting worried, 104–105

managing your, 1

monitoring, 25–26

negative, 91

in panic attacks, 157

positive, 90

realistic, 89, 106–107

separating yourself from anxious, 111–114

taking power away from anxious, 108

visualization of, 60–61

Thought-sensation-behavior CBT model, 67

Tics, 13

Touch as self-soothing, 80

Tracking, 128

Triggers

    of anger, 68, 69, 70

    of anxieties, 23

    external, 19

    internal, 19

    for panic attacks, 163

V

Visualization, 29–30

    combining with abdominal

        breathing, 55

    lake meditation and, 46–47

    as self-soothing, 80

    of success, 153–154

    in teaching mindfulness, 40

    of thoughts, 60–61

W

Worried thoughts, 101

    limiting, 104–105

    reality-checking of, 106–107

Writing in anger reduction, 85–86

Z

Zooming in on negative thinking,
    94

ACKNOWLEDGMENTS

To my girls—Sarah, for your excellent and attentive proofreading and advice; Emma and Hannah, for putting up with me while I wrote and wrote. I love you all and hope you grow up to be wonderful, strong women with solid anxiety management skills. To Yosef, thank you for your moral support, household management, and 11 years of teamwork that allowed me to take on this project during an already busy year in our lives.

To Tonya Swartzendruber, thank you for introducing me to mindfulness and helping me with that chapter. Thank you to my CBT support network for your help with metaphors, skills, and training.

Finally, to my editor Meg Ilasco—thank you for finding me on Twitter and trusting me with this project. This has been a wonderful opportunity to use my therapy skills in a different way, and I'm truly grateful.

ABOUT THE AUTHOR

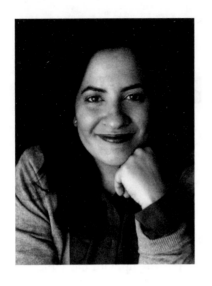

REGINE GALANTI, PhD, is a licensed psychologist who focuses on treating children and teens with anxiety. She specializes in cognitive behavioral therapy (CBT) and has expertise in obsessive-compulsive disorder, anxiety, parenting, and behavior problems. She is the founder of Long Island Behavioral Psychology in Long Island, New York, where she brings warmth, sensitivity, and a tailored problem-solving approach to her practice.

As a clinical psychologist, Dr. Galanti applies short-term, evidence-based strategies to help young people change their thoughts and behaviors. Specifically, she uses exposure and related behavioral therapy techniques to help those living with anxiety face their fears so they can live happier, healthier lives.

Website: **www.longislandbehavioral.com**
Twitter: **@reginegalanti**
TikTok: **@dr.galanti**